"This is a must-read for every one providing the information and to... forming a healthy relationship with food."

—David Meyer | *Fitness Director, Family Ministry Center, Hendersonville, TN, and ACSM-Certified Personal Trainer*

"*The Liberated Eater* changed me from the inside out. I was a self-loathing, bulimic, compulsive eater for over thirty years . . . I still love eating, but I love life more. Food is no longer my boss. I am free!"

—Angie Gregg | *Workshop Member, Writer, Mom*

"This valuable book reinforces the concept that we are all born with all of the intuitive wisdom we need to know how to eat and explains how dieting can lead to a disconnection from that wisdom. Concrete advice is offered to guide you back on the path of reconnecting with that wisdom and to finding peace and satisfaction in eating for the rest of your life."

—Elyse Resch, MS, RD, FADA, CEDRD | *Coauthor of* Intuitive Eating

"*The Liberated Eater* . . . is the perfect read for people who feel out of balance or out of control with food. These truths have caused me to identify the reasons I eat other than hunger and how to trust my body again. I intend to keep this book as a constant reference."

—Eric Stamper, O.D. | *Optometric Physician*

"*The Liberated Eater* is full of profound truths that brought me back to the freedom I knew long ago. Cindy's insight is amazing . . . [with] practical tools that have resulted in lasting, sustainable changes for me personally."

—Kirsten Mickelsen | *Curriculum Sales Advisor*

"Cindy and the information in this book have forever changed my life. At times, food felt like the one thing I had control over until I realized it was controlling me . . . Being a Liberated Eater truly is freedom!"

—Chad Jones | *Workshop Member, CPA*

"Cindy's effervescent spirit infuses *The Liberated Eater* with a tone that is hopeful and powerful, full of encouragement, and laden with powerful tools for enacting the real work of change . . . If you've lost hope in diets and in the strength of your own will to fight the beast of dysfunctional eating, this book is for you."

—Christi Schroader | *Workshop Member, Artist, Educator*

"The information in *The Liberated Eater* will change your life. I know, because it changed mine. I have been liberated! . . . It's full of truth, simple strategies, tools, cutting edge science, and humor."

—Carol Howald | *Workshop Member, Business Owner, Grandmother*

"Cindy has provided timely information in a compassionate, nonjudgmental manner that has been life-changing for me. *The Liberated Eater* will be a treasure for anyone who is longing to have a sane, balanced relationship with the wonderful food God has blessed us with."

—Miriam Frank | *Workshop Member and Grandmother*

"I *loved* this book. Cindy understands how the brain works (hint: willpower *doesn't* work) and has put together an easy-to-understand, powerful process to help people change. *The Liberated Eater* is about food, but it could just as easily be applied to any behavior."

—Dr. Ted Klontz PhD | *Author of* Mind Over Money, *Researcher, Speaker, Trainer, Consultant, Life Coach*

"Cindy Landham has developed a healthy relationship with food, and in this American culture that is a feat. She beautifully shares that journey in *The Liberated Eater* in a fun yet serious manner—rich with data, professional enough to be clinical, and simple enough to be entertaining."

—Kay P. Arnold, NCC, LPC/MHSP | *National Certified Counselor, Licensed Professional Counselor/Mental Health Service Provider*

"*The Liberated Eater* will bring you hope and freedom. I went through her workshop years ago, have released weight, and gotten on with my life. Reading this book brought back so many memories! . . . How thankful I am that this message of recovery came across my path at such a time of desperation."

—Sue Beals | *Workshop Member, Physical Therapist*

"*The Liberated Eater* is an indispensable tool to counteract our harmful cultural messages. Cindy Landham backs up years of research with her simple message . . . a cohesive guide for anyone who wants to emerge from body hatred, food obsession, dieting, and weight cycling."

—Dr. Tracy Tylka, PhD | *Pioneer Researcher of Intuitive Eating, Author, Ohio State University Associate Professor*

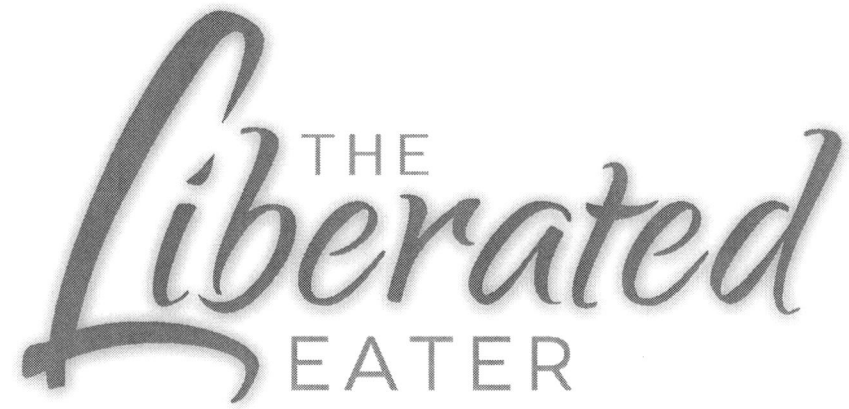

THE Liberated EATER

{ Food Is Not Your Problem.
Dieting Is Not Your Answer. }

CINDY LANDHAM

Publishing Management—Dan Wright Publisher Services, LLC
DanWrightPublisherServices@gmail.com

Editorial—KLOPublishing.com

Typesetting—Katherine@theDESKonline.com

Cover design—VolaciousMedia.com

Author photo—Cali Ashton Photography

Disclaimer: I am a Wellness Coach. Coaching is not meant to take the place of medicine or therapy. If you think you need medical help or counseling please find it and work diligently with these professionals to reach your best health.
If you're experiencing an emergency put this book down and call 911.

CONTENTS

PART III
The Emotional Side of Things
Changing the Conversation in Your Head and Heart

PART IV
Choosing How You Think
It Really Matters

PART V
Rewriting Your Eating Scripts
Changing Those Mindsets and Situations That Lead Us to Overeat

PART VI
Fuel In, Fuel Out
Eating and Playing in Order to Be Fully Alive!

PART VII
Balance—Gotta Have Some
Body & Soul

*To my cherished workshop friends and
fellow sojourners on this liberated eating adventure. Thank you for
your honesty, willingness to share your stories, and courage to
do the new thing—to change. To do things differently.*

*Our lives have intersected at some of our most vulnerable places and
it has been a privilege to meet you there. Your strong desire for truth,
for best health and real freedom draw me forward.
We have changed and are changing still.*

IS LIBERATED EATING A GOOD FIT FOR YOU?

Restrictive/Compulsive Eating Assessment

*J*f you identify with many of the thoughts listed below, you will find the message of Liberated Eating extremely helpful. None of us has to continue responding to food in this way.

If you:

[ ]   consistently find yourself too full after eating

[ ]   have been dieting too long, with little or no success

[ ]   get a little sick just thinking about another diet

[ ]   experience uncontrolled late night or TV eating

[ ]   sometimes eat in secret

[ ]   are often ashamed to eat what you want in public

[ ]   feel guilty for eating "fattening" foods

[ ]   feel angry with yourself for disobeying a food/diet rule

[ ]   don't trust yourself around "fattening" foods

[ ]   think about food way too much

[ ]   turn to food when you are stressed, bored, angry, etc.

[ ]   aren't sure what it means to eat normally anymore

[ ] over-exercise to compensate for eating too much

[ ] think of food as "good" or "bad" depending on its nutritional/fat content

[ ] feel hungry all the time

[ ] feel like you have a food radar; whenever you're around food it is hard to ignore it

If some of these thoughts resonate with you, keep reading . . .

LONGINGS & LIFE STORIES

This book is for the battle weary—those so tired of dieting and dealing with this "food thing" that you've just about given up. If this is you, take heart. It is also for those who have somehow avoided the diet-trap, and perhaps even weight concerns, but struggle with compulsive eating.

You have an invitation to peace—to a relaxed and livable place with food where your mind and body can heal and become strong again.

Most of us feel very alone in the battle even though two out of three people struggle with food. Shame and eating in secret often accompany our disordered eating, and with this comes isolation. Isolation is the last thing we need and the first thing we tend to choose when we're in pain. As we keep these struggles to ourselves, they seem to grow and gain power. We feel frustrated, flawed, confused, and guilty.

Connie remembers the day—the moment—that food and her body became an issue. It was the day she realized she was "unacceptable." She was thirteen, carefree and quite excited about summer as she and her mom went swimsuit shopping. Her mother sat on a stool in the dressing room with piles of swimsuits in her lap while Connie tried them on one by one. She was daydreaming about swimming at camp when her mom said with a tone of disappointment, "I wish you'd gotten my body instead of my sister's. You have her big bottom."

With those unexpected words everything changed. It was as though the curtain parted between childhood and adulthood, between being carefree and being self-conscious. A dark door opened for Connie and she was shoved through it. She remembers looking in the mirror with new and unfamiliar eyes. Eyes that saw flaws and shame. There was no going back to the way it was before.

Not everyone has such a defining moment but many of us can relate to feeling shame over body and food—to believing that something is terribly wrong. Please hear this. This is not your fault. You are not broken. And you are not alone in your behaviors or feelings. If you've tried everything, have spent way too much time and money on "losing weight," if you eat to cope with emotions, if you've ever eaten half a pecan pie in seven minutes while hiding in the bathroom, or hit the bottom of a new two-pound bag of Reese's Pieces, if you've sworn you'll never overeat again only to turn around and overdo it at your very next meal, please know you are not alone. This kind of behavior is shared by millions of us, and there are very good reasons why.

Chuck's childhood was always shadowed by his father's serious illness. There was love in their home, but the weight of the constant sickness and the ever present threat of losing his father were always hovering. The sadness and anxiety made food the perfect place to find comfort. His mom was distracted and his older brother was trying to fill his daddy's shoes, so Chuck often had time alone. Food was a faithful friend, a thorough distraction and a quick comfort.

Rick grew up in a family of people who struggled with their weight. Food was a constant topic of conversation, his family's top priority and favorite entertainment. Every family function revolved around food. As he grew up he noticed that this was not true for everyone. He longed to be different—to be stronger, faster, more agile, less encumbered, but he also felt guilty for wanting to be different from his family whom he loved.

The truth is, none of us would choose to struggle with food. There are forces at play here that have nothing to do with willpower or self-discipline. There is the unavoidable backlash of years of dieting that works against us psychologically and biologically. There are cultural influences, our personal story, our family of origin, and our own temperaments that have influenced our path.

Randi never struggled with her weight until her first pregnancy. It was as though a switch flipped in her brain and body. She has not been able to shed the baby weight and has put on more with the birth of each child. As a stay-at-home mom, a calling she cherishes, she finds it is easier and easier to isolate herself.

Tim is a successful business owner, loving husband and father, and active in his church and community—but almost every night he is overcome by a force which feels greater than himself as he eats large amounts of food, alone, after his family goes to bed. He feels helpless, confused, and ashamed.

Allison was energetic and athletic growing up. She didn't think much about her body or weight. As she grew through her teenage years, she experienced some minor weight fluctuations but certainly nothing that bothered her. It did, however, bother her parents. Rather than changing their minds or having an honest, forthright conversation about their concerns, there were years of hints, innuendoes, unspoken tension, and vague remarks. Food became a power struggle—the elephant in the room. The result has been anger, confusion, and mistrust—and a very strained relationship with food, body, and parents.

It is easy to see how each of these people came to struggle with food for very different reasons. For each one food could mean something different—comfort, a family bond, a distraction, a forbidden treat, safety, power and independence, a way to cope with emotions—no matter what the details, controlling food has become a major issue.

Here's the good news: there are clear and livable answers for each of us. No matter how long we've struggled, we can find the freedom we long for. This book and the resources it will point you to will give you the help, tools, insights, strategies, and message you need to find your good and healthy path to freedom with food and your body. Look for the special icon 🗙 for behavior-changing tools. Other strategies and "thought resources" are not specifically marked.

As you read through this book, you'll gather information, insight and the encouragement you've needed to build a new relationship with food. I invite you into peace. Your food fight can be over.

Sharing My Story, and Hoping to Hear Yours

I remember food and me getting along just fine, and I like to think of those days. I was a typical kid growing up in a small Southern town in the 1960s, riding bikes down Bagley Drive, catching lightning bugs, playing outside with the other neighborhood kids after dinner till our moms called us home—no thought of my body being unacceptable or food being important.

> One of the biggest tragedies of the whole diet culture is not just what we focused on but what we missed.

My mom had struggled with her weight for years. When I was in the fourth grade, she successfully lost sixty pounds. It was 1967; the year my dad was in Viet Nam. Like the rest of us, just because Mom was slim didn't mean that food and weight were no longer an issue for her. And if it was an issue for her, it was going to be an issue for me, because she wanted to save me from the agony of being overweight.

Eventually puberty took the place of childhood. The 60s morphed into the 70s. My body and the times changed.

Food became a frequent topic of conversation. The beloved milk I enjoyed at dinner became taboo. Food became good and bad, fattening and not fattening, legal and illegal. Teen magazines came on the scene with plenty of pictures of long-haired, thin girls in bell-bottoms and midriff tops. There were countless articles on diet and exercise. Food, weighing, thinness, cottage cheese, boiled chicken, grapefruit—these became the focus of my life and many of my friends' lives as well. This was the beginning of America's obsession with dieting.

One of the biggest tragedies of the whole diet culture is not just what we focused on but what we missed. What was squeezed out by the endless food/body conversation and preoccupation? And the ever present weight chart which was to be magic motivation to get me to the pinnacle of all existence . . . weighing 124 pounds. These charts, by the way, were continually replaced by the next one. I don't remember ever actually reaching the goal. They were put up with great hope and then abandoned and replaced and abandoned and replaced.

As food and weight became more and more of a life-focus, my relationship with it and my body became more and more disordered. Mom played the
role of the food police and my dad, who is a physician, got in on it too. I am
sure they were just as frustrated as I was! They had perfectly reasonable diet
plans and check-in points that should have worked like a charm—but I was
unable to comply. This approach, as well meaning as it was, led me to obsess
about food, sneak to get it, overeat it, lie easily and creatively, to feel ashamed
and confused about my behavior and yet continue to do it. I felt helplessly
out of control all the while desperately wanting to be thin. It was a perpetual,
exhausting cycle of trying to restrict intake, breaking the sacred food laws,
bingeing and then—utter despair and shame. Inevitably there was the false
hope of the next new diet that was going to do the trick this time . . . and then
. . . another failure. Exhausting!

I went to college in the fall of 1975. I was in "control mode" at the time
and hit the beautiful Auburn campus weighing 124 pounds. The food police
were far away. There was pizza anytime and cookies to help me study. By the
end of my first quarter I weighed 165 . . . maybe more. I refused to weigh
myself after that. I was mortified to go home to my family, so during the last
three weeks of the quarter I ate nothing, drank Tab and instant coffee, rarely
slept so I could burn calories day and night, and went home wired and *almost*
acceptable.

Laxatives, "water pills," fasts, and drastic exercise plans defined my
restrictive, controlled self. Industrial sized honey buns, Fritos and M&Ms
chased by Dr Pepper defined my out-of-control-self.

My weight fluctuated wildly during those years. Falling in love proved
to be a good appetite suppressant, so by the end of college I thought I had it
under control. As Bob and I married and began our life together, I had times
of temporary food sanity interspersed with the old crazy place. I had begun to
walk or run a few miles a day in college, which kept the weight swings down
to twenty or thirty pounds rather than forty or fifty. But here's an interesting
truth—the amount of weight didn't matter. It was the *issue*—the torturous
thoughts, the preoccupation with food and body, the shame and confusion
of compulsive eating.

When I look back in my journals, I am exhausted by the recurrence of
the same theme over and over again—the burning, all-consuming desire to
be free.

Finally in my early-forties, something happened. I was sitting at my desk making, yet again, another weight chart to go on the back of the bathroom door when a voice in my head caught me up short. "Who are you kidding? How many of these have you made? You're never going to change."

I sat there a minute in light of this revelation. So this was hopelessness. This was resignation. I couldn't do it. I couldn't change. This was never going to work, and I had finally faced it. But oddly, with this revelation I felt strangely giddy.

I decided right then and there that I was never going to diet again. Never! I tore up the chart and ceremoniously threw it away. I thought I should feel a deep sense of failure, but instead I felt some freedom even though I feared the unknown.

I resigned myself to the fact that I would gain weight until I died. That would be sad, but I just couldn't endure the thought of another diet. So that was the way it was going to be. I did promise myself two things: First, I would stop *big* bingeing. Since no foods would be illegal anymore what was the point? I could eat what I wanted anytime now. And, second, I would keep walking most days because I knew it kept me from getting depressed. This was my new life.

Months later I realized that I had not really gained much weight. A year later I realized that I had actually lost a little. A few years later I realized that food was not on my mind much anymore. In fact, it was almost in a relaxed place. Just making it all legal did something incredible for me. Removing the law—the failure and the inevitability of shame—let some intuitive things naturally fall back into place over time.

I became very curious about what had happened to me. How had I grieved and struggled through thirty years of dieting and gotten nowhere and then given up entirely and found a relatively peaceful place with food? This didn't make sense!

As a teacher and a curriculum developer for twenty-five years, it was natural to begin to research the subject. I talked to sane eaters and insane eaters, doctors, nurses, fitness trainers, professional dieters, those who had lost and regained many times, and the few I could find who had lost and not regained. I studied change and why it happens for some and not for others. I earned my wellness coaching certification during this time and learned a world of great information from my instructors at Wellcoaches Corporation.

As my file began to thicken, a few things became clear . . . and then a few more. There were common threads that ran through the research and the stories of people who made real lifestyle changes that stuck.

This freedom was starting to make sense. What had happened to me wasn't a fluke and was actually something anyone could learn and develop. This was too exciting to keep to myself; I had to share it! Liberated Eating Workshops were born out of this passion to share such good news.

Since then, I have learned much from my fellow sojourners. We each have our own story, our own dreams and longings and our own unique way of living with food. But there are some common proven truths that we can all trust to lead us away from a place of disorder to a place of peace and liberty with food, with our bodies, and with ourselves.

This book is simply the natural next-step of our Liberated Eating Workshop community. Those of us who have traveled this path together often speak of passing it on and are excited to share the freedom we've found and are continuing to develop. You will find many real-life stories on The Liberated Eater Web site. It would be an honor to hear yours. If you would like to read more stories or share your own, please visit www.theliberatedeater.com and click on "Sharing Our Stories."

Throughout this book you will read some recurring themes and phrases. We are more likely to make true life-style changes if we hear things more than once in sixty thousand words. And some things have more than one application; you will see what I mean.

Keep in mind as you read that Liberated Eating is not a subject that can be covered in quick sound bites. It is a life-sized concept. Please read through to the end so some very important elements will not be missed.

As I began to write, Kyle, my editor, said these life-giving words, "Don't complicate this. Just write a love letter." So I wrote the reminder below and read it every day before I began to peck away on my computer . . .

Remember why it's important to write this book:

- To bring help and hope to many who feel helpless and hopeless.
- To awaken the original confidence within us that we can indeed hear and honor our body's messages—so we can get and stay well.
- To reinstate the understanding that getting well and being well is as natural as breathing—even in this loud and distracting world.

- Because people are missing their good lives while being preoccupied with disordered eating. There are joys to share, trails to
hike, games to play, paintings to paint, missions to accomplish,
fun to have, gardens to plant, books to write, people to meet . . .
too much good living to be done NOT to write this book.

With all my heart I believe that each of us can find the freedom we long
for. We can learn from the past, look forward to the future, and live fully in
the present.

PART I

Side-Tracked

Starting Well,
Then Getting Knocked Off Course

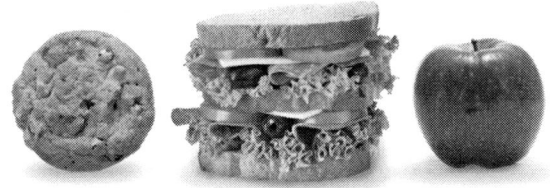

Chapter 1

SANE EATING— IT'S IN YOUR DNA

You were born free

*I*f you've picked up this book, you and I have something important in common. We share an earnest longing for freedom . . .

- freedom to live peacefully with food
- freedom to live comfortably in my own body
- freedom to trust myself and my body and to live in sync with it
- freedom to be in my right mind in any food situation
- freedom to think about living rather than eating

The first thing I ask when I meet a new friend on this journey is, "What's your story?" I am spellbound every time. There are so many ways and reasons that we have been knocked off the "normal eating" path. Every person's life is fascinating! Some of us have simply lost connection with our intuition through years of dieting. Some of us have very specific events, experiences, and even trauma that have shaped our relationship with food and body.

One thing is very encouraging: each of us (barring rare health issues) was born with a balanced and healthy food relationship and we can have it again. It's in our DNA. We were born eating in a way that was peaceful and effective for our amazing baby body and mind. We felt hunger and began to squirm and cry until someone fed us. While we ate, we concentrated on the satisfying experience of getting that warm life-giving milk into our bodies. When we felt "just right satisfied" we turned our head and that was that. We were done. And then we didn't think about food again until our little body needed more fuel and let us know.

It really was that simple, and it worked beautifully. We were all born with a strong inner wisdom to know how to fuel ourselves, with no anxiety over whether or not we would get it right. Don't we long for that again? Freedom to live peacefully with the body you have right now is possible. No matter how crazy you've felt, you can find your sane place with food again. No matter how hard you've struggled, the war *can* be over. I know after years of struggle this can sound too good to be true. But it is true. In fact, living well with the good gift of food is your birthright.

As surely as your body helps you get a reasonable amount of air, sleep and water, or tells you it's time to visit the restroom, your body will help you find a reasonable balance of fuel for your optimal health. Your body is talking to you all the time. You may be out of practice when it comes to hearing what it's saying—but you will certainly be able to resurrect the naturally intuitive eater[1] in you.

Not long ago I was having this conversation with one of my workshop friends. After a lifetime of dieting one month and gorging on sweets uncontrollably the next she never dreamed she could relax and be at peace around desserts. She had just helped with a baby shower and was rejoicing that she had thoroughly enjoyed one delicious piece of moist vanilla cake and was perfectly sane and satisfied—wanting no more. She walked out to her car afterward so grateful for her freedom. I hear these stories all the time—liberty is possible!

> No matter how crazy you've felt, you can find your sane place with food again. No matter how hard you've struggled, the war can be over.

Let's look at some very important things to acknowledge as we begin this journey.

You Are the Expert on You

You know yourself better than anyone else on the planet. Let yourself grasp how powerful this is!

Diet rules and the resulting disordered eating may have damaged your confidence—but this is redeemable. You are perfectly capable of finding and keeping your best health and a comfortable weight. Begin to entertain the thought that getting well and staying well just might be as natural as breathing for you.

We live in a time of many experts on every subject, each one proclaiming they have the answer you need. But people rarely follow expert advice even after they've paid dearly for it. Why? Because we don't own it—the expert does. Certainly we will carefully consider information given to us but for you to move forward into the wellness, energy and freedom you want—you have to know that ultimately only you can make the best choices for yourself and you have the power to follow through. You can and you do.

One of the most exciting things about this non-diet approach to living well with food and body is that we each discover our own unique ways of eating and moving. We each find what works best for our mind and body, therefore we can keep doing it without great effort. Some people end up eating six times a day. Others find they feel best eating twice a day. Some love to hit the gym five times a week and others have no formal exercise regime but are quite fit. Some people find great clarity in journaling their feelings about this journey and some would rather eat a slug than write anything down. Only you can know what is beneficial to you and what is not.

Become the expert on you that you already are. Take charge of your path. You were born with the wisdom to take excellent care of yourself.

You Can Accomplish What You Want to Accomplish in Spite of Obstacles

This may sound unbelievable right now, but it's true. You can accomplish what you want to accomplish regarding your health, in spite of obstacles. Begin to practice saying this. Begin to practice trusting this. Believing this for yourself is the most important work you will do.

This is what a good coach knows is true and what I believe about you: You can reach your health and weight goals. Sure, you'll meet some obstacles along the way; everyone does. Some of my obstacles are asthma, hypoglycemia, a tendency toward addictive behavior and a knee that screams if I try to run for long. In spite of challenges I *know* each of us can reach our optimal health—the best health you can have at your age and in your life situation. You're not hopelessly trapped where you are right now—no matter how it feels.

The war can be over. It is very important that you allow yourself to begin to believe it.

My certainty about this is greater than your doubt!

Getting Well and Staying Well Is Doable and Natural

No matter how crazy you feel right now—if you're eating in secret, having a regular late night love affair with green mint chip ice cream or hitting the drive-thru more than you want to admit to yourself—you can have a sane relationship with food.

Getting and staying well is as natural as breathing or walking or waking up. You can do this. Our bodies are built to run well. Natural processes have purpose and life-giving momentum behind them. Let yourself lean into them. I'm not saying that this is going to be "easy as pie." Nothing great is. What I am saying is that eating intuitively is natural work. Dieting is unnatural work. Everything you need for this adventure is in you already. You and your body have a natural wisdom, an inner compass that will surprise you when you give new behaviors and beliefs some space in your life.

The work we will do will not be *extreme*. Extreme diets and weight loss schemes are exciting and promise quick results—but they don't last. We're after real change that lasts. The process of becoming a liberated eater will take time and will be more than worth the journey. Former UCLA Coach John Wooden put it well, "When you improve a little each day, eventually big things occur . . . Don't look for the quick, big improvement. Seek the small improvement one day at a time. That's the only way it happens—and when it happens, it lasts."[2]

Chapter 2

DIETING: A BIG REASON FOR OUR INSANITY

You're Perfectly Sane— It's the Diet That's Crazy

One of our biggest obstacles to finding the freedom we long for is that we've been given an unworkable solution. For the past seventy years or so, if you found yourself heavier than you wished to be, the answer you were probably given was "Go on a diet." I admit that dieting sounds reasonable. It's simple math. The problem is that you are not a mathematical equation. You are a complex creature. In mathematics, when we subtract, the difference is smaller. In human beings—it often works just the opposite. Most of us have actually gained weight over our dieting history rather than lost it.

There's a mountain of data that points to an abysmal success rate for restrictive dieting. Depending on the stats you read, 90 to 98 percent of us gain the weight back within one to five years. Isn't it time to admit that dieting really does not work for us?

Success is getting food and fat off our minds and getting on with our good lives—not dieting the weight back off every year or so.

So, Why Don't Diets Work?

The fatal flaw of restrictive dieting is very simple: Too little food leads to too much food and makes us a little crazy in the process.

Dieting is built on two principles that simply do not work for human beings: *deprivation* and *hyper-control* of our food.

1. In human beings, DEPRIVATION eventually leads to *excess*, and
2. HYPER-CONTROL eventually leads to *obsession*.

These are definitely *not* the things we were hoping to get from our diet.

Problem #1—Deprivation

If I held you under water for sixty seconds, how would you breathe when I let you up? If you were lost in the desert for three days and finally found water, how would you drink? If someone kept you up for two nights in a row, how would you sleep when you finally got in your cozy bed?

When it comes to primary needs, under-doing it leads to over-doing it. When we haven't had enough we want a lot in response.

This is not about willpower, so give yourself a break. It's about physiology and psychology. Our crazy binges have not been about us being weak. They've been about us being human.

Problem #2—Hyper-Control of Food

When we're dieting, we are focused on obeying the particular food rules for that particular diet. We become obsessed with the foods we can have . . . and the foods we can't have. We become obsessed with our bodies— every pound, ounce and inch. We weigh and measure our bodies like we weigh and measure our food. I

> The fatal flaw of restrictive dieting is very simple: Too little food leads to too much food and makes us a little crazy in the process.

know people who get up and weigh in the middle of the night.

Obsessing becomes a way of life. It may feel normal. It is not normal.

We eventually become scale-focused, body-focused and food-focused rather than life-focused. There is an unhealthy self-consciousness that comes with dieting.

We're going to take an eye-opening look at what's been happening to us over our dieting years so that we can understand it, forgive ourselves, and move forward.

Before we do, let's introduce a way of thinking that *will* work for us.

Think a New Way to Live a New Way

Throughout this book we will be fundamentally changing how we think and live. This balanced and life-giving philosophy has been distilled into thirteen Core Beliefs of Liberated Eating which are the essence of our new way of thinking and are signposts on our path.

Feel free to rewrite them in your own words. They are *yours*, not mine. Find the words that resonate with you. Many have found it very helpful to put them on note cards or their screens and have them close by. I have a set by my bed and in my purse. In a culture that does not encourage liberated eating it helps immensely to review them often. You'll also find a complete list in the appendix. I have not numbered them because the order is not important—some will be more impactful to you than others, depending on your circumstances at the time.

 Core Belief

DITCH THE DIETS

I want a healthy relationship with food, not a restrictive one. I do not diet because diets are unnatural, unnecessary and ineffective. Dieting upsets the peaceful balance that is meant to be between my mind and my body.

Peaceful balance—that is where we're headed.

Before we plunge into a sustainable solution for our best health and weight, let's understand why dieting has never worked for us permanently. This will give us confidence to leave the old conventional thinking behind and move forward into a whole new way of living.

Why Diets Haven't Worked for Us Psychologically

Diets make you want what you cannot have. The more you can't have it, the more you want it. Forbidding certain foods causes you to focus on that food. You might rarely want a doughnut if you didn't think you shouldn't eat them. It is the forbidden doughnut idea that makes you want one every time you drive past the bakery . . . especially if the "HOT" sign is on! Making a food "illegal" gives it false power over you.

Diets make food a moral issue because of the good food/bad food rules. This eventually leads to "I'm good" or "I'm bad" according to what I eat. Thinking of food as good or bad makes it seem like an ethical choice when it isn't. You are not a good person when you eat a salad and a bad person when you eat a piece of candy.

Once we believe that all food is *not* the same in moral weight, it becomes difficult to make an honest, unemotional decision about what we really want to eat. "Should" and "should not" changes everything.

Food is not a moral issue. It is neutral. Let this thought begin to bring food down a notch or two on your anxiety scale. (We're not speaking of nutritional value here. We'll get to that.)

Dieting leads to shame. Many dieters feel a great deal of shame. Shame over not being able to stick to a diet. Shame over eating compulsively. Shame over sneaking food and hiding the evidence.

All this says to the dieter that they are broken. There is something wrong with them. They have a terrible secret. They are weak and have no willpower.

Dieters often shame themselves for their appearance and for their failures at trying to change it:

> *Paradoxically, weight loss practices such as restricted eating may amplify the experience of body shame rather than alleviate it. In and of themselves, weight-loss practices lead women to pay more attention to weight and shape, which can heighten and/or increase the frequency of their awareness of their failure to meet physical ideals. Failed weight-loss attempts or an inability to maintain weight loss may also increase body shame. A vicious cycle may then ensue in which failure to meet body ideals leads to body shame as well as weight-loss efforts that may compound the experience of body shame.*[3]

Although these psychologists were addressing the situation of women, in our culture today the same issues are affecting men as well.

Dieting causes anxiety. We're often anxious about being around food that's not "on the diet," trusting ourselves around food, not getting enough food or eating too much food. And since food is a regular part of life, this anxiety is ever-present.

Getting on the scales can be anxiety producing. Feeling judged about our progress or lack of progress can cause anxiety. When we're "being good" we feel anxious about not eating the food we want; when we're "being bad" we feel guilty but are at least eating food we like. Dieting is anything but peaceful.

Diets focus on the negative "I can't eat *that*" is continually ringing in our heads when we're dieting. We are constantly thinking, *I shouldn't eat that* or *This is not on my diet.* All these thoughts remind us all the more that we want to eat those foods.

Diets are not sustainable. Research shows that diets get shorter and shorter the further along we travel along our dieting trek. They get less pleasant and more impossible to handle and we grow less and less confident. No one can live on a perpetual diet and no one needs to.

Dieting causes us to have a sense of desperation and/or entitlement about food. While dieting we are underfed so the food we *do* get to eat becomes entirely too important to us. We eat every bite and want to lick the plate, and heaven help the person who tries to eat a bite of our carefully measured food! After the diet has ended, these intense feelings don't just go away. We still feel we're entitled to the food we have and feel desperate about not getting enough.

The memory of deprivation is deep and powerful and influences our feelings toward food. These feelings have a big influence on our urge to clean our plate. Dieting creates an unnatural anticipation and excitement over food that makes it difficult to stop eating even though our stomach has had enough.

Dieting takes away our liberty, which is a primary human need. Why would parents put their family in a small, rickety boat and take them across dangerous waters to get to freedom? Because we are created with a deep need to be free—to be able to be reasonably self-governed.

Living under diet rules is like living under a dictator . . . we will either rebel or give up eventually.

When dieting is our lifestyle, we give up our freedom to be flexible and intuitive. Diet rules become our authority. It isn't long before we lose touch with the confidence and inner wisdom we were born with that would naturally guide our own health and balanced food choices.

Effective change happens and real freedom comes from the inside out, not from external rules and negative commands pressing from the outside in.

Diets consume precious time and energy. How much life did I waste thinking about dieting, being thin, looking through magazines (which only led to being very unsatisfied with my body), planning the next exercise regimen, preparing the next shopping list and making charts? Then there was time spent thinking about food—what I should eat, what I shouldn't eat, what I want to eat and how I can get it. There was time spent sneaking and plotting about how to get around the food police—not to mention the shame and anxiety this caused.

Dieting sucks life, time and energy from the momentum and meaning of our real lives. It's time to take back those stolen hours and reclaim that wasted energy!

Dieting gives a false sense of control. It provides a temporary sense of control, order and security (at first). Dieting is a powerful distraction from real living and authentic coping. We feel hopeful that *this* diet is going to be the answer to *everything*.

Don't be surprised if giving up dieting may turn out to be uncomfortable at times; the false hope it promises is seductive.

Dieting causes us to eat excessively when we normally would not. Diets *begin* with an eating fest because we have to eat plenty of what we'll "never eat again." Then, when we cannot bear the diet any longer, we end it with another eating fest, enjoying all those wonderful foods that were forbidden.

Since our ability to adhere to diets diminishes over time we can end up practically going from one overeating cycle to the next with little dieting in between.

Dieting can affect us socially. You may become reclusive when you're on a diet so you won't be tempted by foods that are "illegal." Then, you may become reclusive when you're off the diet so you can eat in secret or because you feel shame about eating "real food" in public.

Your personal story can affect how dieting affects you. We all have our own life story, temperament and bent. There are certainly universal ways that the deprivation and hyper-control of dieting affect us as human beings, but there are also personal experiences with dieting that play out in us individually. This quote from *Intuitive Eating* by Elyse Resch and Evelyn Tribole may be helpful to keep in mind as we begin our journey toward liberated eating:

> *"If you have experienced deprivation in areas outside of food—such as love, attention, material needs—the deprivation connected to dieting may be felt more intensely for you."*

Why Diets Haven't Worked for Us Biologically

Deprivation slows your metabolism. This causes your body to burn less fuel than it normally would. This is *not* what we want. Our metabolism is like an engine. We want it to idle high, running through lots of fuel. When we diet our body is concerned about not getting enough fuel, so it conserves. Your body "adjusts down" in order to survive longer on your skimpy diet menu. Remember, your body has no idea you would actually voluntarily decide to starve. Most of our popular diets are considered starvation by the body.

When you begin to eat normally again (or more likely overeat) it will hang on to the extra fuel for the next "famine." You actually can't eat as much as you did before the diet without gaining weight.

To add insult to injury, most of the time we not only lose fat on a diet, but water and muscle as well. When the diet ends we often gain back fat and water only. Muscle is dynamic tissue, burning lots of fuel, so losing it further lowers our metabolism.

The good news is that as you begin to take good care of yourself, your body will begin to recover. Your metabolism will begin to trust you again. Beginning to move, play, and walk more will go *a long way* in helping you rekindle your healthy metabolism. As you become more active it will become more active as well. Take heart!

Frequent fluctuation in your weight and eating pattern is harmful to your health. Studies show that it is healthier to stay a bit overweight consistently (provided you're healthy) and eat more normally than to lose and gain the same weight for years. This is a lot to put your body through.

Consider this: Good health and beauty come in different sizes and shapes. If you and your doctor agree that you are in good health, you could explore the possibility of becoming happy with your weight right where it is, or at least carefully reconsider the "goal weight" you thought you wanted all these years.

Do you feel great? Do you have the energy you want? Are you comfortable in your skin (once you get the waifish media pictures out of your mind)? Only you can know this—but it may be time to stop thinking that "being skinny" is the ultimate meaning of life. Just considering this can be freeing and relaxing.

Dieting goes against your natural biology. It falsely reduces a primary, biological need to a matter of willpower. Remember, human beings are built to obsess about food when they don't get enough of it.

Your body *and* your brain cause you to crave food when you're restricting your fuel by more than about 300 calories of what is needed to maintain your present weight. Most diets take us well below this mark.

After a diet, eating can feel desperately out of control because your body and brain thought you were starving. Too little eventually leads to too much.

Because we believe and have heard for decades that dieting is just a matter of self-control, we think that our out-of-control eating is a character flaw—so we feel weak and ashamed. Please understand: this is about biology and biology always wins eventually. Yes, we do have willpower and self-discipline. We are amazing creatures with amazing capabilities, and we need both of these attributes. But to apply them to you and your primary needs is simply unworkable. Go ahead . . . try holding your breath for three minutes. . . just use that self-discipline of yours.

Air, water, sleep, and food are not matters of willpower. The premise behind restrictive dieting is a complete misunderstanding and disregard for how your body and brain work. Restrictive dieting is like asking yourself to need less air. You would never feel guilty for needing the amount of air your lungs ask for each day.

Dieting Causes Us to Do Crazy Things!

Bottom line, when we adopt a lifestyle of dieting we begin to act in ways that we normally would not—ways that do not work for the good of our mind or body.

Take this familiar scenario: You're on another diet. You're really serious about it this time too. But somehow you find yourself reaching for one of those tiny little Tootsie Rolls in a candy dish as you're leaving the office. As you walk toward your car you unwrap it and eat it.

You taste the sweet wickedness of that tiny Tootsie Roll, and it's wonderful . . . until it's all gone. Then you realize what you have done. You have broken the law! What were you thinking!? The mere thought that you broke the sacred rule sends you into a tailspin. You feel utter disgust at yourself and begin the berating process. This is easy to do as it is well practiced. You travel down the road feeling as though you've just committed adultery. And then you utter those fateful words:

"I've blown it . . . again!"

This "I've blown it" (on a tiny and powerful eleven-calorie Tootsie Roll Mini-Midgee) is utter and complete defeat. Now, we all know what comes after "I've blown it!" After the initial shock wears off there is this strange and slightly euphoric realization that comes over you:

"If I've blown it . . . I might as well . . . blow it big."

When she is good, she is very, very good; but when she is bad, she is horrid. And why not? Law breaking is law breaking, right? Why not do it right.

So, what in fact was an inconsequential eleven-calorie blip on the screen of your day becomes a belly-aching train wreck. There's a Snickers on the way home, double stuffed pizza for dinner and then some ice cream—all the while promising yourself you're back on the wagon tomorrow. Well, actually, Monday makes more sense.

This, my friend, is the *Official Crazy Place.*

You lay in bed that night feeling guilty, regretful, weak, and heavy. You lose trust in your ability to ever be around food. The cycle of law breaking and shame perpetuates itself. And the longer you live in this cycle the farther you get from hearing your body's life-giving messages and the more you believe that you simply cannot behave with food.

Let's think this through: "I've blown it, so I might as well stuff myself!" makes as much sense as saying, "I just got a scratch on my car, I might as well total it!"

You would never think this. You are a reasonable and rational person. You know a scratch is a small thing. It may be disappointing, but it is not nearly fatal. It does not make you go to the crazy place.

Dieting has skewed reality for us. I see this all the time in workshop. I am looking around the table at people I admire. People who raise families, manage homes, go to school, run businesses and organizations and are loyal employees. They vote and don't litter very often. They take care of aging parents and neighbors. I'm talking about the kind of folks that make the world a better place—but they would argue otherwise. Why? Because of this one thing. *Their reaction to food* has got them stymied. They are convinced that they're weak and powerless.

Please hear this truth: You have never failed a diet. They're not work-able. Diets have failed you!

Allow yourself to hear this . . . to actually consider that this could be true. It probably won't sink in the first time or even the second. But this is true scientifically and experientially for millions of people. The verdict is in. The research is clear. The statistics are indisputable.

Diets simply cannot work for the human body or the human psyche. They are indeed counter-productive. In fact, if you know someone who would like to gain weight, you have their answer. Just put them on a diet and in time they will gain weight. Not only will they put it on but after dieting for a while, weight is gained very easily and very quickly. This is virtually foolproof—a 90 to 98 percent success rate!

Here are the results of some studies:

- "After weight loss, the rate at which people burn calories decreases, reflecting slower metabolism. Lower energy expen-diture adds to the difficulty of weight maintenance and helps explain why people tend to re-gain lost weight." June 26, 2012, *Newsroom* article, Study by Dr.'s Ebbeling and Ludwig, Obesity Prevention Center, Boston Children's Hospital

- Dr. C. W. Callaway of Mayo Clinic found that most fad dieters gain back *more* weight than they lose. Drastically reducing calories results in a decreased metabolism rate to conserve energy. This makes weight loss very difficult.
- At the University of Pennsylvania, a group of obese lab rats were put on a restrictive diet. Once their weight was back down to normal they were allowed to eat freely again. It took them forty-six days to regain the weight. After trying the same restrictive diet a second time, it took the same group of rats only fourteen days to regain it.

> You have never failed a diet. They're not workable. Diets have failed you!

We see this in our own lives, don't we? After dieting, it seems that the weight returns easily even when we believe we are not overeating. There are many things at play here. We rarely go back to "normal eating" after a diet. But it is also true that our bodies can and will put on weight more easily after a period of starvation.

As chronic dieters we are doing things to lose weight that are actually causing us to keep or gain weight, not to mention causing us to feel confused, discouraged, and guilty.

Read this fascinating study and let the truth of it sink in; this is *not* about your willpower.

DIETERS AND STARVATION SUBJECTS RESPOND ALIKE

The first in-depth understanding of the damaging effects of dieting was clinically demonstrated in the Minnesota Starvation Study. The findings in this 1944-45 study, led by renowned scientist, Ancel Benjamin Keys, Ph.D., have now been confirmed over and over again by top researchers and by our own life experiences.

In the 1940s starvation was widespread throughout war-torn Europe and very little was understood about it. Dr. Keys and his team conducted the study at the Laboratory of Physiological Hygiene at the University of Minnesota for the War Department. Their hope was to understand the medical needs facing millions of starving people and how to re-nourish them. The study was published in the two-volume, Biology of Human Starvation (Minneapolis: University of Minneapolis, 1950).

40 young men were carefully selected for being especially physically, psychologically and socially well-adjusted. They were put on restrictive diets of about 1,600 to 1,800 calorie per day for 3 months. They dieted to lose about 2.5 pounds a week and to lose 25 percent of their natural body weight, and were required to be physically active. Their calorie intake was higher than many weight loss diets attempted today.

As the men lost weight, their physical endurance weakened and reflexes became sluggish. They felt tired and hungry, had trouble concentrating, were dizzy, had body aches, headaches, and trouble sleeping.

The unexpected psychological changes were astounding and were much like we experience today while dieting. Dr. Keys called it "semi-starvation neurosis." The men became anxious, apathetic, withdrawn, impatient, self-critical of their bodies, moody, emotional and depressed. They experienced feelings of inadequacy and lost interest in their usual pursuits.

As the study progressed the men became increasingly irritable. Their senses of humor and compassion decreased.

The act of restricting food and constant hunger "made food the most important thing in one's life" said one participant. "Food became our obsession" said another.

Several men began collecting cookbooks and recipes. Some began hoarding things, drank large amounts of coffee and tea and chewed gum incessantly. Binge eating episodes also became a problem. Many men developed odd eating rituals to make meals last longer. Some stole food and admitted to eating from garbage cans. Two men suffered severe psychological distress resulting in brief stays in the University psychiatric hospital.

The aftermath: When the men were allowed to eat at will again, they had insatiable appetites, yet reported never feeling full. The men were warned to be careful not to eat too much too soon but many couldn't resist. Even five months later some continued to have disordered eating.

The men regained their original weights plus 10 percent. The regained weight was disproportionally fat and their lean body mass recovered much more slowly.

Does any of this sound familiar? Please recall that these men were specifically chosen because they were physically, psychologically, and socially well-adjusted. These were not weak-willed men.

No one can diet and act normally toward food. You tried valiantly but it simply could not be done. You didn't fail. You are not weak. You, my friend, are a perfectly normal person who responded as a perfectly normal person is supposed to respond to food deprivation.

As this reality begins to sink in, consider, just consider, allowing yourself to stop blaming yourself and have some compassion for you and others who have traveled this impossible road. Now, let's turn our faces forever toward a new way of thinking and living with food.

Take a deep breath and imagine your life without dieting. No more counting, weighing, planning, adding, or subtracting. No more guilt over broken food rules. No more going places and being afraid about what kind of food will be there—or not be there. No more restricting, telling yourself you're not hungry when you are. And no more deprivation, which is one of our major binge triggers.

Let's leave what hasn't worked behind and embrace what will.

So If Diets Don't Work, What Does?

Your body is on your side. You can trust it. Taking your cues from it will help get you to your best health. You're probably very intuitive about listening to your bladder, your fatigue and your thirst. You don't really think about them until they get your attention. This leaves you free to live your life.

We have already mentioned how babies are born as intuitive creatures. They sleep when they're sleepy. They poop when they're poopy. They eat when they're hungry. They stop when they're satisfied. Babies are very intuitive because no one has had time to convince them to over-think things yet. They do what comes naturally.

Eating intuitively causes them to thrive. Because they are prompted by their body's messages, they have plenty of energy and time for other important things.

Each of us was born eating in this relaxed way—and we can live that way again.

Core Belief

LISTEN TO YOUR BODY—YOU CAN TRUST IT!

I can trust my body. It is built for high performance. It knows what it needs, when it needs it and how much. I pay close attention to my body's signals, such as hunger, fullness, thirst and fatigue, and I honor them.

This way of living is so freeing! Once you get used to it you'll wonder how you ever lived otherwise. Think about this: what are you focused on when you're dieting? Food. What are you focused on when you're overeating? Food. But, when you are eating intuitively you are *free* . . . free to focus on life, people, work, play, learning, exploring, thinking, doing that thing you've always wanted to do.

This is way more fun than thinking about your next snack!

Liberated eaters are free to get on with living because they trust their body to tell them when to eat. It's like having an alarm clock you trust. You can relax and sleep, trusting it will tell you when to get up.

So, how are we going to make this happen? We're going to continue to develop new *Core Beliefs*—beliefs based on what is true and effective. We're going to rediscover our *Core Behaviors*—the behaviors that we were born with. And we are going to become masters of proven tools that can get us through any eating situation with confidence and sanity.

PART II

Finding Our Path to Freedom

Becoming a Mindful, Intuitive and Informed Eater

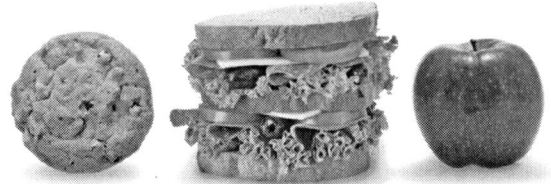

Chapter 3

KNOW WHO YOU ARE

You Were Born to Live Peacefully with Food

There are many different reasons we have fallen into a frustrating relationship with food. And, because we live in a time when we're barraged with conflicting information about *how* and *what* and *when* we should and shouldn't eat, many of us are confused and overwhelmed to the point of giving up. This is understandable.

I've read I should eat every two to three hours to keep my blood sugar stable and that my stomach must be empty five to six hours between meals. Diet drinks are a good way to keep my calorie count low—and they will put me in an early grave after frying my remaining brain cells. Whole wheat seems to be the best choice and the cause of many health problems.

Sheesh! Not only do we have information-overload, we have *conflicting* information over-load.

We can certainly discuss the science behind all of these statements, but that isn't the point—the point is that this is confusing. And, to complicate things further, all this information comes from experts.

I get frantic e-mails and calls regularly from people who just want to get and stay well, but the information swirling around in their heads is making it very difficult to find a clear and confident direction. Couple that with the fact that most of us with dieting histories don't trust ourselves anyway and we can become an anxious mess!

So what do we do?

Like so many things in life, the answer is simple but profound. Know that you were born eating beautifully for your own health and well-being. You are the expert on you. Only you can know what your body is saying to you and how it responds to the way you are feeding it.

Yes, it is important to be reasonably informed—but information is not *wisdom* (and our information is subject to change). You and your body have your own wisdom. You can relax and trust it. Our goal now is to become mindful, intuitive, and reasonably informed—and to relax and enjoy living this way.

Let's take a closer look at the direction we are taking:

- *Mindful*—peacefully connected to yourself and the moment, attentive, observant, present, aware of how you are responding to food and your body. This is the opposite of mindlessly eating on auto-pilot or being unaware of what is going on in your body and mind.
- *Intuitive*—instinctive understanding, using your inborn wisdom, in-sync with your body's messages, insightful. This is the opposite of being disconnected from your body's signals while blindly following arbitrary diet or exercise rules.
- *Informed*—Having a reasonable, relaxed, practical and workable knowledge of food and your body. This is the opposite of either staying uninformed or becoming anxious, overwhelmed or perfectionist because of information overload.

Bottom line—we were born living peacefully and healthfully in our bodies. If we had never been convinced otherwise, we would still be doing so. We were created to be fully alive—not to stress over food, exercise or our bodies. They are meant to be *lived out of*—not obsessed over.

> We were born living peacefully and healthfully in our bodies. If we had never been convinced otherwise, we would still be doing so.

Obsessing over our bodies and food is like having an awesome car and never enjoying it. I'm not talking about my twelve year old mini-van here. I'm talking about a brand-new midnight blue convertible sports car. Amazing! It's built for high performance and tailor-made with *you* in mind. It fits like a glove. The interior is made to order for your particular needs. It's built for the road—built to put down the top and to cruise down the road with you feeling the sheer joy of driving! This is one great machine.

Suppose I rarely take her out on the road. What if, instead of taking her for a spin every day, I sit in the gas station and fret about gas and oil and antifreeze and tire pressure. There you'll find me sitting at the pump week after week pouring over the gasoline choices . . . there's unleaded and high-test and premium. There's Shell and BP and Exxon and the 7-11. Which should I choose? What can I have? Which one is best? What catastrophe will happen if I choose one over the other? This is very confusing and the more I obsess about it the more anxious I get. Since I'm too anxious to listen to my common sense, some days I pump way too much gas and other days I ration it out in a pinched fashion seeing just how little I can get by with. I laser-focus on scrutinizing the body of my car and find multiple flaws. I compare my car with the others that come through the station.

I could put the top down and take off under the sun with the wind in my hair and "Born to Be Wild" blaring from the speakers—enjoying being alive and on the road! Instead, I fume and fuss over the details of my car but rarely enjoy it.

This feels like a terrible waste, doesn't it? You're thinking, *let ME have this car—I'll show you what to do with it!*

When we're absorbed with dieting, bingeing, food rules, pounds, inches, the number on the scales, exercising, not exercising—when our relationship with food consumes us—we are missing the ride of our life when all we need to enjoy it is right under our nose.

Listen, you don't have to miss the ride of your life. You don't have to be sidelined while everyone else lives their life (at least that's the way it looks). You can *live!* Yes, it may take a while to implement some changes. You may have weight to release—and thoughts to renew—but you can do it! You are free to drive with the top down.

• Chapter 4 •

KNOW WHERE YOU'RE GOING AND WHY

Creating Your Own Wellness Vision

*J*t is very important for us to firmly know, without a doubt, where we are going with our health and why we want to go there.

Dan and Chip Heath put it this way in *Switch: How to Change Things When Change Is Hard,* "The people who change have clear direction, ample motivation, and a supportive environment." As you read this book, you are in a certain place with your health, weight and energy. You feel a certain way in your body right this minute. I'm assuming that you're not happy where you are. I'm also assuming that you probably have some idea where you wish you were. For many of us this has been solely centered around a number on a scale. We think if we could just weigh X amount we would be happy. This hasn't done the trick so far so let's change our approach.

It's time to create your personal *wellness vision.* That's a coaching term for a vivid and compelling mini-movie in your brain that you can quickly access anytime. This is the picture you can pull up when you see warm donuts in the break room but you just had a good breakfast and aren't the least bit hungry.

This wellness vision is you on your best day. This is you—the way you want to feel and look and move and dress. This is you feeling strong and free and vital, doing what you love to do. This is not a goal you reach and then forget. This is your life. What setting would best represent this longing for you? Strolling along the beach, hiking in the woods, playing with your kids or grandkids, traveling, dancing at a wedding? You decide and begin to let a powerful vision form in your head. To keep it top-of-mind you can write this down, draw a picture, find a film clip—whatever captures your vision in a way that keeps it fresh. This is *for you!* There is no right or wrong here—just you finding an enjoyable and compelling way to describe where you're going . . . your health destiny.

My best friend, Bob the intuitive eater, was proofreading through this section of the book for me and said, "This wellness vision thing is powerful!" As we discussed why, it became clear that he had formed a wellness vision without realizing it. He envisions himself doing the things he loves to do—being able to hike, paddle, climb—nothing hindering him from what he enjoys. This love of outdoor adventure keeps him from doing things

> Wanting things to be different *and choosing to do things differently* are not the same thing.

that might jeopardize it. This is a powerful force for his health—for living in a way that keeps him fit. He loves a good cigar and a bowl of ice cream as much as the next person, but he loves being well *more* so he lives in a balanced tension with all these good things.

The Importance of Importance

It's essential for you to know how *important* reaching your wellness vision is to you because wanting things to be different and *doing things differently* are not the same thing. How important this is keeps you on the path of change even when you want to get off, gives you the will to live a new way in the middle of an old pattern, keeps you getting up after having fallen down for the umpteenth time. Deep longing gives us courage.

A very effective, self-coaching tool for clarifying the difference between what we *think* we want and what we *really* want is the 1 to 10 Scale:

Use a scale from 1 to 10, 1 being "not important at all" and 10 being "*very* important." Here's how it might play out for me—the cookie monster. Let's say I just had breakfast and am completely satisfied. I don't need any fuel right now. I end up at a meeting where there are very yummy looking cookies. If I feel a strong urge to eat a cookie I can use the scale to help me decide what is most important to me. I step away from the table, take a few deep relaxing breaths and ask myself two questions: On a scale from 1 to 10 how important is eating a cookie to me right now? I'm not hungry but it still *feels* like a 9 (keep in mind I have a long history of cookie lust). On a scale from 1 to 10 how important is it to me to feel fit and peppy? I discover that I want the cookie on a 9 but I want to live in my wellness vision on a 10. I find my chair and turn my thoughts to the meeting at hand. Peppy wins. The 1 to 10 scale can clear up confusion. And by the way, I can take a cookie with me in case I want it next time I'm hungry.

Here are some questions that will help you figure out how important reaching your wellness vision is to you:

- What will be different for you when this goal is reached than it is today?
- What will you have then that you don't have now?
- What will you do then that you don't do now?
- What will you enjoy then that you don't enjoy now?
- Why is this so important to you?
- Who or what will this affect?

You have just described your wellness vision and now have a pretty good idea of how important it is to you. Hang on to your dream. Consider it your destiny. Review it often. Get excited about it! Make it more and more vivid.

Understand that in a world of yummy, ever-present, abundant food, you gotta want your best health like a parched soul wants water, like a blind man wants his sight. You gotta want this more than you want cookies in your mouth.

You have to do the work of deciding if you want your dream more than you want the things that are keeping you from it. Yes, it's okay to want those cookies—we just have to want to be well a little more. This is very important to know and this is why it's imperative to have your vivid wellness vision ready. You never know when you'll need it.

Chapter 5

WHAT YOU CAN EXPECT ON THIS JOURNEY

Clear Expectations Are Powerful

S ince I stumbled into my liberation about twelve years ago and now have had the high privilege of traveling alongside others making the journey—some things have become clear. Though we all have our own unique stories, there are some mile markers along the way that most of us encounter.

When you're on a journey, the idea of expectations is huge—knowing what to expect along the way stokes your anticipation, keeps you encouraged, and pulls you forward when you're ready to quit. Let's take a good look at what we have to look forward to, and what to be prepared for between where we are and where we're going.

Several times a year we visit Bob's family in Griffin, Georgia. From north of Nashville to south of Atlanta can feel like a pretty long trip, and when the kids were small we heard, "Are we there yet?!" often. If we broke the trip down into "legs of the journey," we didn't hear it quite as much. Somehow knowing we were going from home to Interstate 24, from 24 to Chattanooga, from Chattanooga to Atlanta and then from Atlanta to Griffin just felt more doable. The boring parts were more tolerable and our anticipation more keen as we saw ourselves getting closer and closer to Monner's house.

This trip to resurrecting the Liberated Eater in you is much like a road trip. At times you'll think you should be there by now! If you have some idea what to expect, it's easier to hang in there when your patience wears thin.

Of course no two people will experience this journey in the same way exactly. Change is not a straight line. It's organic, multidirectional, messy, and often includes many different emotions. As with any journey you will experience exhilaration and deep contentment as well as some frustration, ambivalence, and inner resistance. Embracing every new day with a sense of curiosity and flexibility is imperative.

> For true change to happen, the pain of staying where you are has got to be greater than the pain of changing.

Stepping back into old ways at times is not failure; it's a normal and important part of true change. With this in mind, let's get started.

As terrible as it sounds, this road to recovery usually begins with misery. And this is a good thing because for true change to happen, the pain of staying where you are has got to be greater than the pain of changing.

Often the first leg of the journey looks something like this:

- You're completely worn out. You've tried it all and nothing has worked long term.
- Shame and hopelessness have settled in. You feel like a failure and can't muster the strength to try one more diet.
- You may hate your body—or at least feel betrayed by it.
- You don't trust yourself with food—especially "fattening" food.
- You're not sure what it even means to "eat like a normal person."
- Your quality of life is directly affected by this struggle. It is an ever present drain.
- Maybe you're even frightened by where this weight/food thing is taking you and your health.
- You desperately want to be free of this struggle but think it's no longer possible; to say you're discouraged is an understatement.
- The thought of listening to your body feels foreign, and you haven't a clue what hunger or satisfaction feel like.

Then you hear about a completely different way of approaching this problem—can there actually be a way to get what you want without dieting? You're cautiously willing to consider the possibility that this just might work. You've tried everything else. What have you got to lose? You let yourself feel a tiny ray of hope again and decide to give this non-diet approach a try.

The second leg of the journey goes something like this:

- You begin an intentional pursuit of freedom—stepping out of the old ways and into the new.
- Eating mindfully feels odd and hyper-conscious at first.
- Giving up dieting feels exhilarating—and scary.
- You and your body start to patch up your relationship with each other—you begin to work on trusting and listening again.
- You begin to think more about *how* and *why* you're eating instead of *what*. This may feel counterintuitive—even dangerous—but freeing.
- Permission feels scary since diet-rules have long been your norm.
- You may choose formerly "forbidden" foods often on this leg of the journey.
- Nutrition may be off balance for a while. This pattern will not last, but you must walk through the permission stage in order to restore food to its proper and sane place in your life.
- You find that you're reconnecting—becoming more conscious of what your body is saying to you about your hunger, your food preferences, and your fullness.
- Freedom with food feels awkward and elusive.
- The thought of relaxing with food and letting your body lead feels too good to be true—but you see it working and catch real glimpses of freedom.
- You may be concerned that this is too relaxed, not structured enough. Dieting had such knowable boundaries.
- You may feel impatient because weight loss is not as fast as it was when you were restricting food.

As you practice this new way of living you notice some wonderful things happening. The next leg of the journey looks more like this:

- You see that the more satisfying your eating experiences, the less you think about food all day.
- You begin to find your personal food likes and dislikes. Some things surprise you. Many of them are nutritious foods.
- Waiting on true hunger begins to feel more normal and very satisfying. You actually prefer it.
- You're beginning to learn to respect your fullness. It's difficult at first and you'll still overeat some while in this learning process,

but you learn to give yourself mercy instead of punishment when this happens.

- The old nagging diet mentality begins to slowly die.
- You are building relaxed, pleasant food experiences. The more experiences you have, the more you believe in your ability to make this change permanent.
- Your hyper-focused preoccupation with food lessens.
- Choosing satisfying foods becomes easier.
- You begin to trust your right to choose and your ability to hear your body.
- You start to feel more peaceful and less anxious around food.
- There's less sadness when a meal ends because you are beginning to trust that you can always eat when you're hungry.
- It takes less food to satisfy you.
- You can often tell true hunger from emotional hunger now, and you are much more likely to find real solutions to emotional discomfort.
- You begin to release weight more consistently.
- You experience an increased sense of well-being.

Somewhere along the way you will begin to realize that your old dysfunctional way of living with food has given way (most of the time) to peace and freedom. How long this will take depends on your story, diet history, focus on this process, and how consistently you use your tools—but you will arrive. Home is just around the bend as you start the last leg of your journey.

- All your intentional work comes together into a comfortable, easy eating style that is all your own.
- You actually prefer to wait on true hunger and stop when satisfied because you feel so good in your body and don't want to jeopardize that.
- You begin to choose lighter, healthier foods because you feel great when you do.
- You truly believe no food is forbidden. "Special" foods do not have power over you. You can enjoy them thoroughly, but it doesn't take much to satisfy you completely.

- There's no more urgency—the knee-jerk reaction to deprivation is gone.
- You're less afraid to identify and deal with emotions—rather than stuffing them down with food.
- Your inner voice and conversations are positive and peaceful.
- You respect your body. Weight loss naturally happens (if it needs to), your body finding a comfortable weight, and fluctuation ends.
- You can't stand to use food for anything other than what it is.
- Nutrition and exercise are completely different to you now. Moving feels good. Choosing and eating life-giving food feels good. You're not operating from "should" anymore—but from a place of "want to."
- There is exhilaration, hope, and expectation about your health. You feel younger and more vital.
- You feel empowered and no longer susceptible to outside forces and influences.

Let me encourage you to return to this chapter often. It will remind you where you're going and why it is so worth it. When you're in the middle of a struggle, it is easy to forget.

When frustration and condemnation are loud, come back here to regain your bearings. Remember where you're going and that it will take time. Sometimes you'll run. Sometimes you'll walk. Sometimes you will even fall. When you do, just fall forward.

You are doing good work, brave sojourner, and you are on the road that will take you where you've always wanted to go.

Chapter 6

KEEP THE MAIN THING THE MAIN THING

Choosing a Dream Strong Enough to Change Things

J really want to lose this weight!" How many times have we said it, cried it, prayed it, screamed it? But it just isn't enough, alone.

For a time you will need to take the goal of releasing weight off the "Most Important Thing in the Whole World" list. (I like to use the term *releasing weight* rather than *losing weight* because we tend to find what we lose. When something is released, it's given its freedom and not expected to show up again.)

Now before you shut the book, hear me out—it doesn't mean you will not release weight, many do so immediately, but it does mean that it can't be the only and main thing. Weight loss—that magic number on the scale we think will bring us all the bliss we've ever wanted—has been the main thing for a long time, and it hasn't worked well for us, has it?

Think it through . . . if you drop weight but haven't learned a new way of living with food, the weight will come right back as soon as the effort is over. If your relationship with food hasn't changed, then sooner or later you will go back to your old way of living with food. It is impossible to do otherwise if something new has not taken the place of the old. I understand. I spent thirty years losing and finding the same pounds over and over again.

As long as being thinner or reaching a certain number on the scale is our *only* goal, we will not be able to release weight and keep it off. Yes, being thinner will feel great—and for many of us it's an important part of being well—but it can't be the only thing we desire.

You might be thinking, *Why not? You don't know how badly I want this! I want to be thinner! I want a new body, dang it! And I want it now!* Well, what's new? We've wanted that for a long time, but *wanting that* hasn't changed a thing. We're still wanting it and we're still struggling with food.

> *Reality Check:* **Being thin is not the holy grail.**
> Thin people feel miserable and suffer
> from depression as often as overweight people do.
> Yes, being thinner will feel great.
> But it is *not* the answer to all your problems.

Wanting to see one certain number on the scale is not getting you any closer to your goal.

Angela was going to a big family wedding. People she had not seen in years would be there, and she determined that she would look great. She set a goal of 130 pounds and worked hard to get there. She reached 140 by the big day. She definitely looked like a million dollars and knew it. Her husband said so and so did many others. She had a blast the entire weekend! But here's the interesting thing—because Angela was focused on the number 130, she felt like a failure. Never mind that she felt great, looked great, and did not need to weigh 130 pounds—in her mind she had failed. Once the distraction of the wedding was over, she began to berate herself for not reaching her goal weight and gained back every pound.

It wasn't until she came through workshop that she put two and two together and realized the folly of being scale-focused instead of life-focused. Her intuition and body told her that she was gloriously content. The arbitrary number in her mind convinced her otherwise.

Let's rethink this thing . . . completely. The thought of you at the magic number just doesn't stick in the face of warm brownies or hot, cheesy pizza, does it?

You know that old saying "Nothing tastes better than thin feels"? It's a lie—at least in that moment. I can tell you right now that when I'm faced with warm, homemade chocolate chip cookies, they look yummier to me *right then* than the thought of thin feels *right then*. There must be something more important than thin.

You must have something firmly in place that carries more weight than just losing weight. You need a rock-solid motivation . . . an immovable anchor . . . a supreme purpose that will hold when you don't even want it to hold. This is your *wellness vision*—your health destiny—the idea that's driving your bus. This is what you ultimately crave *more* than any warm brownie.

Being honest with yourself about the food you crave and the health you say you want is crucial. Once you're clear about what you want most, you can do the work of developing a relationship with food that will drive you toward wellness, not through the drive-thru.

This is, after all, what motivates "normal" eaters. They don't want to eat past full even though it still tastes good. Why? Because it doesn't *feel* good to feel bloated, sleepy, heavy, and slow. Intuitive eaters like the taste as much as anyone, but they will not jeopardize feeling great just to have more of what they've already had.

Everything must be ultimately driven by this: *I want to be fully alive. I want to be well—really well, in my mind and body.*

 Core Belief

BEING WELL IS THE GOAL

I eat, drink, play, work, move and rest in a way that causes me to be well. My goal is to thrive, rather than weight loss alone.

This is our new reality, our truest and highest motivation. Of course you may still want to be thinner—and that's great—but this weightier desire must be even more firmly in place.

When your greatest desire is wanting to be as well as you can be for as long as you can be, then you begin asking the helpful questions that will take you where you want to go.

If I just want to get skinnier then I'm asking questions like:

- How many calories, fat grams or points are in that?
- Is this fattening?
- Is it "bad" for me to eat this?
- What kind of exercise torture must I endure so I can have some?
- If I starve the rest of the day, can I have a piece?

> Everything must be ultimately driven by this: *I want to be fully alive. I want to be well— really well, in my mind and body.*

These kinds of questions are not life-giving. They are pinched and small and leave us feeling deprived. We get very tired of living under them.

People who have a balanced relationship with food don't have these kinds of thoughts in their head. People who live well with food and are comfortable in their body ask different kinds of questions:

- What's going to hit the spot? Which of these choices "jazz" me the most right now?
- Am I in the mood for smooth or crunchy? Warm or cold?
- What's going to make me feel great—now, an hour from now, a day from now, and a year from now?
- What's going to feel satisfying in my mouth and in my stomach?
- What's going to give me the energy I need for the next four or five hours?

These questions may be asked subconsciously because they're intuitive. These thoughts are promising, invigorating and life-giving. These thoughts make room for good food and good life.

Chapter 7

MOVE FORWARD IN YOUR RIGHT MIND

Being in Your Right Mind Requires Being Mindful

There are only a few things that set "normal eaters" apart from the rest of us. These things are simple and have nothing whatsoever to do with dieting or restricting. This is where we want to go. Let's look at them . . .

FOUR CORE BEHAVIORS OF LIBERATED EATERS

1. They eat when they're physically hungry (not emotionally hungry).
2. They choose what they would like to eat with both pleasure and health in mind.
3. They connect with their food, enjoying the eating experience.
4. They stop eating when their need for fuel is satisfied.

So, that's it. Nothing drastic. They don't meticulously think about counting calories or being "good" or "bad" or "should" or "shouldn't." They trust their body to tell them when to eat, what to eat, and when to stop. Eating this way is relaxed, peaceful, and refreshing. They are naturally well-fueled—not too little and not too much. This gives their body energy for the day and leaves their mind free. It keeps their weight at a comfortable place too.

None of this stuff is hard or complicated—we can do this! Countless people have gone from compulsive, restrictive, anxious eating to a relaxed and healthy relationship with food. This is a journey we can make.

In case you're wondering, we will certainly get to the subject of emotional eating, but for now let's gain a good understanding of how the health-giving lifestyle of mindful eating works.

> To resurrect the liberated eater in you, you will first need to begin to reconnect with your very wise body.

Interview a Naturally Intuitive Eater

To resurrect the intuitive eater in you, you will first need to begin to reconnect with your very wise body. Interviewing an intuitive eater or two is a great way to discover some very interesting things about this lifestyle. (Good luck finding one, because there are only about one in four of us, but they do exist.) Ask any questions you may have, including these:

1. How often do you think about food?
2. Do you ever forget to eat? (*If they say yes to this, resist the urge to hurt them.*)
3. How often do you weigh yourself?
4. Do you ever feel anxiety over your body, food, weight?
5. How do you know when it is time to eat?
6. How do you know it is time to stop eating?
7. How often do you eat too much?
8. What do you think when you eat too much?
9. Do you enjoy eating a meal? Why?

This is an interesting exercise and very revealing! Have fun with it.

Reflection: What did you learn from your interviews? Which part of the intuitive lifestyle do you look forward to most? Which part seems impossible right now? What answers surprised you?

Chapter 8

RECONNECTING WITH YOUR AMAZING BODY

Listening for Hunger and Satisfaction Again

Hunger is a natural and vital message, but as dieters we have been trained to ignore it. The good news is that it's still there; we just have to learn how to listen again.

[It is very rare, but there are cases where a person cannot hear their hunger signal well, temporarily or permanently, because of bariatric surgery, side effects of medications, etc. They can learn to use other signals and other tools to find and keep their heath. A wellness coach, dietician, nutritionist or health professional can help with this. Remember, every situation is workable. Anyone can improve their health.]

Hunger—Eating for All the Right Reasons

Dieting has skewed our feelings about, and ability to recognize, true physical hunger. We fear or dread it because no matter how hungry we are we can't answer it except according to the diet we are currently on. Or we love it, because it means our body is "eating up that dreaded fat," so we don't answer it. Either way, *hunger* is not being used for what it is. The hunger signal is very simply a natural message from your body telling you that you need fuel for energy. Period.

Where Does Hunger Happen?

Hunger doesn't always feel the same, but as you get to know your amazing body again you will get better and better at understanding what it's saying to you. You can feel hunger in your stomach, head, and limbs. Sometimes it's a core feeling of emptiness. You may feel weak or shaky as your blood sugar drops. You may get a headache or become confused or irritable when you get too hungry.

What Affects Our Hunger?

Certainly when we last ate. But *what* we ate will affect it as well. If you had a Pop-Tart (with little protein or fiber) for breakfast, you will probably be hungry again soon. If you had a handful of almonds with it or opted for two eggs and grainy toast, the protein and fiber will satisfy you much longer and you might just make it to lunch without feeling hungry.

What and how much we eat affects when we will be hungry again (more on this in chapter 24), but there are other factors that can affect hunger as well:

- activity level
- health issues (physical, emotional, or spiritual)
- sleep—quality and amount
- thirst can be mistaken for hunger
- medications can affect hunger and satiety
- stress
- emotions
- diet mentality
- food allergies
- thyroid issues
- hormone changes
- bariatric surgery can affect how you hear hunger and satisfaction
- overconsumption of alcohol, which slows metabolism
- insulin resistance
- diabetes
- leptin resistance
- hypothyroidism—a medical condition that causes weight gain and a loss of appetite
- depression

There are many things that can affect our hunger. This is why it's important for us to become reacquainted with our body's messages. As we learn to
hear accurately we won't often be confused and misled.

Your body is speaking throughout the day to keep you balanced, but as
restrictive (too little) and compulsive (too much) eaters, we have trained
ourselves not to listen. We've ignored true hunger and fullness. We've
ignored what our body has asked us to eat in order to feed it diet food, and
then, when no longer dieting, we've ignored what it really wanted so we
could fill up on all the foods we couldn't eat while dieting.

Your job now is to tune in and learn to hear well again, as you did when
you were a young child. Your mind and body will begin to feel peaceful. Soon
you will wonder why you ever lived any other way and will simply avoid anything that jeopardizes that good feeling.

> Checking in before you dig in will save you a lot of unsatis-fying eating experiences and unwanted weight.

Think of it as if you and your body are
in counseling right now. You are learning
how to communicate and trust each other
again. It's going to be a great partnership!

Let's look at a tool that will help us in this listening process. Try it right
now and then use it often before thinking about a meal or snack. After some
practice this will become second nature. Please understand the importance
of this action—it's the vital first step to eating in a way that is going to get
you the health, energy, and weight you want.

CHECK IN BEFORE YOU DIG IN!

Before you decide to eat—be still a moment. Breathe deeply and let
yourself relax and become aware of your body. Try to shut out any
distractions. If you've had a frenetic day, it may take a few moments
to connect with the sensations of your physical body.

Tune into your stomach. Make a fist, which is about the size of your
stomach, and put it right up under your breastbone. That will help you
locate your stomach and become more aware of it. Now take your fist

away and concentrate on your stomach. How does it feel right now? What is it telling you about what you need or don't need? Is it slightly empty, empty, or very empty? Is it still satisfied from the last time you ate something? Can you feel it at all? If your stomach is perfectly satisfied, you will probably not be able to sense it—it's not telling you anything. It's happy and can be left alone for now. If this feels foreign, don't worry. With practice you will do this very quickly and accurately.

Tune into your feelings. What are you feeling at this moment? Do you feel rushed, distracted, worried, excited, bored? Do not judge your feelings. Just notice them. They will have an effect on how and why you eat. For example, if you're feeling hurried, you may eat in a hurry and barely notice that you've eaten. By the way, if you're truly physically hungry, you may not need to do this at all. You will *know* it. I like what Geneen Roth said in *Breaking Free from Emotional Eating*: "Being hungry is like being in love—if you're not sure, then you probably aren't." Be patient with yourself. It takes time to tune back into your body after years of telling yourself not to listen to anything but what the diet tells you to do.

Checking in before you dig in will save you a lot of unsatisfying eating experiences and unwanted weight. Too often we eat on auto-pilot. We eat because it's dinner time; we eat what we don't want; we eat more than we want; and our eating experience is not very satisfying.

Checking in is vital. If you aren't hungry when you *start* eating how will you know when to *stop*? Eating when you aren't hungry is like scratching an itch that you don't have. How would you know when to stop scratching an itch that isn't itching?

HUNGER/SATISFACTION SCALE

Another tool for getting a handle on your body's health-sustaining messages is to think about your *hunger* and *satisfaction* as being on a scale from 1 to 10. This is simple but very effective in helping you hear the nuances of your hunger and satisfaction.

HUNGER/SATISFACTION SCALE

1. **Starving!** [Shaky, faint, totally depleted—almost impossible to eat mindfully at this point.]

2. **Very hungry!** [Wilted, grumpy, significant lack of energy.]

3. **Too hungry to want to eat at a reasonable pace.** [It's possible but will take intentional effort]

4. **Ready to eat—healthy hunger.** [Eating here is just what your body needs.]

5. **Gently satisfied.** [I could eat more, but am not hungry—this is just right for slow, permanent weight release.]

6. **Just Right Full.** [I can feel the food in my stomach but am not overly full—this is just right for weight maintenance.]

7. **A few bites too many.** [A tad uncomfortable—this is perfect for slow weight gain.]

8. **Uncomfortable.** [You feel too full and have to loosen your belt.]

9. **Very uncomfortable.** [You're tired, slow, beached.]

10. **So full you could barf.** [Even lying down hurts!]

Notice how the reasonable places are toward the middle of the scale—4, 5, and 6. You see words like *healthy*, *gentle*, and *just right*. People who live peacefully with food stay in this range most of the time. They're mainly driven by inner cues so when they get hungry they feed themselves. When they feel that just-right-full feeling they stop feeding themselves. This isn't hard since food is not an emotionally charged issue for them. It would not make any sense to keep eating and then be uncomfortable. An intuitive person wants to feel energized by their meal and ready for the next part of the day.

Now look at the two ends of the Hunger/Satisfaction Scale—these are the *extremes*. You see words like *too* and *so* and *very*. This is where I stayed when I was dieting. I was too often between 1 and 3 while on the diet, and then once "I blew it" I would hover between 7 and 10.

Whichever extreme end you find yourself on, you can almost bet that another extreme will follow—extremes beget extremes! If you let yourself get to 3, which is too hungry to want to eat at a reasonable pace, you will be prone to dive in and eat quickly because you're famished. The end result, more times than not, is that you will eat your way right past satisfaction. It's an interesting thing, if we start eating at a 2, we'll often eat to the same place on the other end of the scale—an 8 or 9. We respond to extremes in the extreme. Same thing with overeating. We often decide after we've overeaten that we need to devise some kind of deprivation such as swearing off sweets for a month, etc. And the pendulum swings.

One of the foundations of a balanced relationship with food is that it's reasonable. Reasonable is sustainable. Extreme is not. Extreme solutions have never worked for us and they never will. Human beings just don't do well with extremes over time. They feel exciting, but they don't deliver.

Our goal now is to begin to tame the swing between the two extremes and start to live more and more in the middle of this scale. We will be listening for physical hunger and answering it by feeding our body when it needs fuel. We will be listening for a satisfied feeling as well. When we feel it, we will begin to honor our body's "done" signal and get up and get on with our day.

No one does this perfectly, not even "normal eaters." It isn't possible or necessary to "eat perfectly." And please be careful not to turn this useful tool into a rigid rule. It can be tempting since most of us are so used to obeying diet rules.

Our new paradigm shift:

- Rules—we break them eventually, then regret it (the Eve Effect).
- Tools—we can use them to build useful things that last.

Tools work better than rules when it comes to living well with food. The real goal here is to get back in sync with your amazing body so you can get well, stay well, and enjoy being well. One of our most important questions becomes: "Does my body need fuel right now?" Or put another way, "Am I physically hungry?"

When we begin to answer this question honestly, and honor it, other things naturally begin to fall into place.

 Core Belief

WAIT FOR TRUE HUNGER

I listen for hunger and answer it, because that is when my body needs fuel. If I eat when I do not need fuel, my body has to store that food as fat.

Notice that last sentence from this Core Belief: If I eat when I do not need fuel, my body has to store that food as fat. This is an *Immovable*—one of those things that we cannot get around no matter how hard we try.

Food Is Fuel—Potential Energy

Food is much more than just fuel to us, but when it comes to releasing weight it helps to understand this truth: food is fuel. Fuel is potential energy. I'm no scientist, as my high school teacher can attest, but I do remember something about energy being constant. It can change form, but you can't create more or destroy it.

This is a very helpful concept to remember when it comes to food. A cookie does not go into my mouth, get chewed up and swallowed, and that's the end of the cookie. It is potential energy. It has to be used as energy or stored. If I'm not in need of fuel I can't use it so it changes into fat tissue. Every Nutter Butter peanut butter cookie will be used to move me around . . . or it will change form and find its way to my hips. Simple.

A 55-year-old woman who is 5'6", enjoys walking 4 times a week for about 45 minutes, and feels best at around 145 pounds will have to take in the amount of fuel that her age, gender, height, and activity level needs to maintain that weight. There is no getting around that. If she eats less, her clothes will get looser. If she eats more, her clothes will get tighter.

We must—and we can—make peace along the way with our *Immovables.* In the next two chapters, let's take a look at:

1. how true physical hunger differs from cravings and urges, and
2. how we can stop eating when we are satisfied instead of continuing to eat.

Getting a firm grip on these two subjects will be key in helping us find and keep the health we desire.

Chapter 9

CRAVINGS, URGES, AND TRUE HUNGER

How Can I Tell the Difference?

True hunger usually builds gradually and occurs three to six hours after your last meal. You want and need fuel. When you want a very specific food *right now* (think Oreo Blizzard) you're probably experiencing a craving, not true hunger.

Cravings are usually very taste-specific and nothing else will do! They may feel strong and urgent or they may nag annoyingly. They're almost always stimulated by external cues or uncomfortable emotions. This is imagined hunger in your mind—disconnected from the true needs of the body. Here's a craving check for you when you're feeling this way: If you would not be happy with a piece of fruit, you probably are not physically hungry yet.

Cravings will usually pass in fifteen to twenty minutes or when you get busy doing something else (get outside, brush your teeth, breathe deeply, take a walk, brush the dog, call a fellow mindful eater, play some music and dance a bit). Just about anything will break the spell, but know this: When a craving jumps on you and threatens to wrestle you to the ground, you are in a critical place in your mindful eating journey. Every time you don't feed the craving but wait on physical hunger:

- you strengthen your improving relationship with food
- you build confidence
- you weaken the power cravings have over you

The next time you feel a craving, tell yourself, out loud if you need to, *I don't have to feed it. It's not real!* It's a bossy craving triggered by a sight or smell or feeling—but it's not real physical hunger.

Decide now that you will *tolerate* the overwhelming urge to eat. Get comfortable with being uncomfortable for a little while. Understand that even though it feels big, refusing it will not hurt you—but giving into it will. This is the perfect place to crank up your wellness vision and play it over in your head a few times. Remember what you really want. Your dreams trump an old pesky craving anytime! When you feel pressured to give in to your cravings, talk it down. Have an inner dialogue ready such as this to talk yourself through:

> *I am not physically hungry right now. When I am, I will eat exactly what I want. This is not deprivation. This is sanity and freedom. I'm in charge here.*

You really start to *win* at this point. Celebrate every victory! Do a victory dance, high five somebody (they don't even have to know why), put a notch on your belt—acknowledge your strength and grit. And give yourself mercy when you need it.

When we starve cravings—they eventually die. Good riddance.

Urges are a little different from cravings. They are intense and short lived, kind of like a firecracker. They last about four minutes and lose half their intensity in sixty seconds. If you keep walking and don't grab that donut, within a few minutes you won't even remember you wanted it. But if you eat it, you will remember and regret it for hours.

> *Norma was walking through the kitchen, not thinking about food at all, when she spied her peach cobbler on the counter. (I should add that Norma is an exceptional cook.) When she saw it, the urge jumped on her! She remembered our conversation in workshop about urges—was skeptical but decided to test it. If it wasn't true, she was going to dig into the cobbler. She set her kitchen timer for four minutes and went to answer e-mails. Later she heard the timer go off and was puzzled. She couldn't remember having anything in the oven. The urge for cobbler was so far out of her mind that she had to think a minute before she could remember why she had set the timer.*

Urges and cravings are wimpier than you think. Get fierce about refusing them. You can eat every time you're hungry now. No more restricting. No more rice cakes or plastic cheese (unless you love them). For us to reach our health goals, waiting for true hunger is key—which makes putting cravings and urges in their place a very important thing to do. And we can.

{ When we starve cravings— they eventually die. Good riddance. }

Here's some really exciting news: As your relationship with food normalizes, and it will, cravings will become less and less intense.

Waiting on hunger is the logical *beginning* of an eating experience. Let's take a good look at the logical *end* of our eating experiences—stopping at "just right" satisfied.

As you read the next two chapters on satisfaction, keep in mind that the chapters that follow will center on what happens *between* hunger and satisfaction. Each intuitive step supports the other—it just takes a while to say it all. Read through this whole section and the pieces will begin to work together nicely.

Chapter 10

FINDING AND STOPPING AT SATISFACTION

It's So . . . Well . . . Satisfying!

*J*ust think about *satisfaction*. What a beautiful word! What could be better than being satisfied? And who wants to be dissatisfied? Yet for those of us who struggle with food, eating can be very dissatisfying: eating too little while restricting, feeling anxious about what we're eating or not eating, eating too much, feeling sluggish and heavy, eating in a hurry, hiding food, eating in secret, gulping down big bites, hearing self-criticism in your head, feeling guilty . . . we could go on and on.

Eating is something we all have to do several times a day, so if much of it results in an unsatisfying experience, it wreaks havoc on our quality of life. This is no way to live. Let's get a vision for how it can be.

I asked some of my friends about their thoughts on satisfaction now that they have been on this journey for a while. Here are their thoughtful responses:

Beth—*The "just right" place" is so comfortable and energizing. My body now tells me when I am there. If I happen to miss it, I can always eat something later on if I want to. I find if I eat when I'm hungry and till satisfied during the day, I am not too hungry at dinner. After dinner I'm happy and done for the day.*

Cynthia—*The amazing thing for me now is that I actually get up from the table and feel light in my body. Where I used to feel a lot of confusion and shame about eating I now feel mostly free and grateful. I just didn't know that was possible. I look back on all those stuffed, sleepy afternoons and wonder why I ever lived that way!*

Carl—*Satisfaction feels like pure freedom! The problem for me was never eating too little. Once I was able to realize, as simple as it may sound, that I could eat more later if I was still hungry, I felt free to experiment. Now I am mindful and present when I eat so I am able to listen to my body—not my empty plate—to tell me when I am satisfied.*

Melissa—*Stopping at satisfied is a good feeling that even goes beyond the comforting feeling of having something I really enjoyed in my tummy. It's the feeling of being in charge. Eating to "just right" feels doubly satisfying to me.*

This kind of food-life is worth fighting for. All these people were plagued by compulsive overeating, feeling defeated and desperate about their relationship with food. They struggled to believe that they could ever have a normal relationship with food. In this chapter and the next we will discuss the understanding, tools, and strategies we need to truly be able to enjoy our food and also enjoy stopping at satisfied.

As with hunger, dieting has affected our ability to hear our satisfaction cue. When dieting, we weren't listening for satisfaction because there wasn't enough food to satisfy our needs—and that taught us to eat every tiny morsel and lick the plate! This deprivation experience installed emotionally charged feelings about food and eating, which only led to more plate cleaning and less and less listening to what our body had to say.

The good news is that our satisfaction signal is still there; we just have to learn how to hear it again. We are about to reconnect. Now as we begin to do the good work of changing our minds, our responses, and our feelings, here are some important points to keep in mind:

Remember that your resistance, fear, rebellion, or current inability to stop at satisfied is perfectly normal. Please reread chapter 2 if you are not convinced that, for those with a diet history, these are natural responses. Of course there may be other factors that drive you to eat past full, such as uncomfortable emotions, being told to clean your plate as a child, not eating until you're famished, eating food that isn't satisfying, or feeling that you can't "waste" food or money. Often these things just add fuel to the fire of our diet-deprivation behavior.

The physical and psychological fear of starvation is powerful and primal. Imagine how upset you would be if you weren't getting enough air. Not getting enough food or water is the same thing, just not as immediate. Dieting has messed with our deepest core! We can certainly straighten things out again, but we must understand that it is going to take time, compassion, effective tools, courage, and support for us to recover the liberated eater in us. That is what we are about.

Believe that you are free. You really do have complete, no-strings-attached permission to eat (or not eat) anything you want, whenever you want. This is critical to you being able to stop eating when you are no longer hungry.

I know this sounds dangerous—but the best things are. Grace is dangerous. We can abuse it. But if we really aren't free to choose it or reject it, then it isn't grace at all. And love is dangerous. If we are forced to love, it isn't love. Love, by its nature, must be volunteered. So where is all this deep stuff going?

> Overeating only feels good while the food is in the mouth. It never feels good later. Regret trumps the thrill.

Bottom line—you have to know that you are free to choose whatever you want to choose. Then—and only then—are you free to choose well. And you can.

It makes sense to want to feel better—not worse—when you're finished eating. It is intuitive to want to feel good—and to avoid things that would jeopardize it. One of the things I love hearing most is the excitement people express as they begin to leave some of their meals feeling light in their body and mind—free to go live their good lives not weighed down with too much food in their belly and the regret that comes with it. After a few of these experiences it gets easier and easier to leave food behind and to trust that you can indeed eat again when you are hungry again.

When we do happen to eat past full, it is a great reminder that overeating only feels good while the food is in the mouth. It never feels good later. Regret trumps the thrill of excess. When this happens, see what you can discover about it, have mercy on yourself, and move on.

Listening for, acknowledging, and honoring your body's messages are sure ways to feel great. When you eat because you're physically hungry, choose food you enjoy and then savor it fully, and stop eating when your body is well-fueled, you're practically guaranteed to feel good.

Stopping at satisfied is a HUGE part of getting and keeping the health and weight you desire. All the elements of this mindful eating lifestyle are important, but everything changes when we no longer overeat regularly: our health, emotional well-being, weight, pants size, energy, what we spend time doing and thinking about. Much of our heartache has come from overeating.

I often hear people on this journey express their enthusiasm about now having room in their life for other things—things that mean so much more to them than overeating ever did.

If releasing weight is part of your goal, the point at which you feel "gently satisfied" is key. This is number 5 on the Hunger/Satisfaction Scale (see Chapter 8), which is just under your maintenance fuel level, number 6.

To hit this gentle satisfaction, eat what you want when you're hungry and be mindful of ending your meal just before full. This is that place where you're not hungry any more even though you could hold a bit more. Certainly this does not have to be done at every meal, but the more often it happens the sooner you release weight.

Eating to this place works because:

- It does *not* cause you to feel deprived.
- It does *not* slow your metabolism.
- It does *not* scare your body or brain into making you prowl for food.

WOO YOUR LEPTIN

If we *rarely* stop when our body asks us to, our leptin, the hormone which tells us we're satisfied, stops saying much to us—like a person who isn't listened to. It can take a few months of reasonable eating for your "I'm satisfied" signal to speak up again, but it will.

Another way to get your leptin to be loud and clear is to get enough sleep. "When you don't get enough sleep, it drives leptin levels down, which means you don't feel as satisfied after you eat. Lack of sleep also causes ghrelin levels to rise, which means your appetite is stimulated, so you want more food," explains Michael Breus, PhD, director of The Sleep Disorders Centers of Southeastern LungCare in Atlanta.

You can be confident that you can do this. You already stop at satisfied in other areas of your life. You can do it with food too.

Begin to think of living with food as you live with other necessary things, such as air, water, sleep. Most of the time your body stops at "just enough."

Think about this logically—which is not how we've been thinking about food, since dieting made food an emotional issue. This is how we operate with our other primary needs:

- There is a prompt from your very smart body, which is managing your systems for you so you're free to go live your life.
- You "hear" the prompt of thirst or fatigue and don't question it.
- You honor it by getting a drink or some rest.
- When the need is satisfied, you stop. You don't keep drinking water. You don't stay in bed (well, usually).
- This feels satisfying. It brings peace, health, and balance to your mind and body.
- You're ready to go . . .

. . . *until it comes to food!* Because of dieting deprivation, uncomfortable feelings, and perhaps our own life story, food has become more than fuel to us. Whether it's become a companion, entertainment, a secret pleasure, medication, a safe place, a habit, or any other thing—it is not simply fuel, and this is where the struggle comes in. We'll talk more about this in Part III, "The Emotional Side of Things."

THE POWER OF MERCY

Here's a big deal to grasp right here and now: While you are prac-
ticing this new skill of listening for and honoring your satisfaction
signal, you will need to have abundant mercy for yourself.

When you've overeaten and feel regret, the next step is kind-
ness. Only then can you move on. Mercy keeps us from getting stuck
in a dark place and gives us the hope and freedom we need to learn
from the experience and move forward.

Judgment and self-criticism keep us stuck like a truck spinning
its wheels in deep mud. Forgiveness sends us on our way.

Know this up front: *You will not do this perfectly and that is not
failure.* No one makes a significant life-style change without missteps
along the way. Relapse is school. Stumbling, getting up, dusting off
your knees and walking on is the very best way to learn.

The life-giving power of mercy is essential for this good work of
change.

Chapter 11

STOP TRYING TO OUT-THINK YOUR BODY

Ignore the Distracting Conversation in Your Head

Your body's primary objective is to keep you running at high performance. It knows what you need in order to be well, and because it doesn't want you to under or overeat, your body will prompt you in many ways to help you stay efficiently fueled.

Fullness can be different for each of us, but there are some common feelings. You might become more aware of your stomach's fullness, you might realize the pull toward food has lessened because your fuel need has been met, you might feel nothing at all because the "wanting" of hunger is over. I often feel just a slight short-lived tightness in my stomach even when I have not overeaten. We will talk more about this in Chapter 15, but realize now that your body is talking to you.

Your mind, however, will try to override your body with thoughts such as these:

- *Oh, just finish that up; there's not that much left anyway.*
- *I paid for this. I need to get my money's worth.*
- *When will I ever get this again?*
- *How can I possibly throw all this food away? It's wasteful!*
- *I'm too stressed to think about this today. I'm just gonna eat it.*

- *Hmmm, I haven't eaten in four hours. I guess I need a little something.*
- *Oh, forget it . . . it's a holiday, the weekend, a new restaurant, a birthday . . .*

Your mind can come up with all kinds of convincing reasons why you should eat and keep eating. These reasons may be compelling in the heat of the moment, but they will lead to regret. The whole time your mind is trying to get its way your amazing body is sending clear messages of exactly where it wants to take you. Replay your wellness vision loud and clear, and do what your body is telling you to do. Just do it—without question. Don't listen to your mind. Don't even give yourself time to think about *not* doing it.

Establishing this Core Belief is a life, weight, and health changer.

 Core Belief

LISTEN FOR "SATISFIED" AND HONOR IT

My body knows how much food it needs. The right amount of food is very satisfying. I often pause halfway through my meal to "listen" for satisfaction, and I stop eating when my body tells me I am no longer hungry.

Like any skill, hearing and answering your satisfied signal will get easier and easier as you practice. The truth is, we are very capable of stopping at satisfied. Recently I had a great conversation about this with Chad, who has been on his mindful eating journey for almost a year now, and he shared this:

I would rather be home than sitting in some hotel room, however, there's one thing I have always loved about traveling on business: the company pays for all of my meals and the choices are endless.

I was recently away on a business trip. This was my first trip after reclaiming my status as a mindful eater. To say that I was a little nervous would be like saying that the Grand Canyon is a little crack in the earth. What was I going to do without all of my safeguards? At home, I'm set for success. My fridge is full of healthy things I enjoy. People at work know

I'm working on being more healthy. Now here I am in a city with no one else, it's dinner time, and I'm really hungry. Thankfully, I remembered to bring my tool box.[4] It's always with me, it only requires that I use the tools in the box.

Tool 1: I remember that the cook does not have a clue about me or my fuel needs. Just because food is put on my plate doesn't mean I have to eat it.

Tool 2: When my meal is brought out, I immediately ask for a to-go box and put some food in it if I feel I'm over-served. Out of sight, out of mind.

Tool 3: This was my favorite, and I may have to trademark it. I took a picture of the food I was served and then, afterwards, what I left on my plate. I have a folder on my Kindle that's titled "Food I Didn't Eat" and I put the pictures there. This reminds me of how I want to feel at the end of a meal before it ever starts, helps me celebrate what I do not consume, and proves how good it feels to leave the restaurant satisfied rather than miserable.

The photo tool is brilliant—so easy and highly motivating. You can just hear the thrill of victory! And by the way, Chad has released twenty-five pounds—and as good as that feels, he is most excited about the peace he now has with food.

As you practice, you will notice that you're beginning to eat from freedom rather than from compulsion. You'll find that you are relaxing into a more enjoyable way of being with food as you begin to believe you really *can* eat when you're hungry. Becoming mindful, listening to your body, using the tools—all these things will begin to come together to pay huge benefits that reach way beyond just releasing weight.

When you dare to consistently stop at satisfied, amazing things happen:

- You begin to trust yourself
- You begin to feel confident
- You begin to have more energy

- You begin to hear and trust your body's signals again
- Your brain chemistry and blood sugar begin to normalize (over-eating is a drastic thing to do to your body and brain!)
- You begin to work with—and not against—your body
- You begin to lose your food anxieties
- You begin to release weight
- You begin to relax around food and in all food situations

We have *a lot* to look forward to!

Tools for Finding Satisfaction

Here are some effective tools for honoring your satisfaction cue:

 Best Bites First

Go ahead, treat yourself luxuriously! Eat the very finest bites first from now on. Look at the food, smell it and then decide what looks the very best to you. Enjoy each wonderful bite.

I used to save the best bites for last, and I know I'm not the only one. But think about it. To save the best for last practically guarantees that I'm going to eat everything on my plate, even the yucky stuff. I hate to think of all the stale bread and cold mashed potatoes and burnt edges I've endured so I could eat those sacred last bites.

Eating the best *first* is a very reasonable thing to do—and you're allowed to do it. The cool thing is that it becomes very easy to leave food on your plate when all the best bites have already been enjoyed.

 Two-Minute Mid-Meal Pause

This is simple and very effective. About halfway through your meal, *pause* for two minutes. Stop, put down your fork or food, sit back, relax, breathe slowly, take a few sips, and *check-in*. Feel for satisfaction.

This is a speed bump. It's not necessarily a call to stop, just to slow down so you can see where you are. Fast-paced eating momentum makes it too easy to zoom right past satisfaction.

For you musical types, think *metronome*. Any of us can start a meal at a mindful waltz but within six bites be up to heavy-metal-head-bangin' scarf speed without even realizing it! The Two-Minute Mid-Meal Pause helps you reset the tempo to "adagio."

Be open to the possibility of being satisfied. If you are, you are free to be done. If you are not, go for the very best bites of what's left. We will talk more about this in Chapter 14.

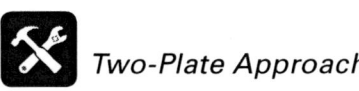 *Two-Plate Approach*

> The skill of Mindful Eating is like any other skill—the more you practice the better you get at it and the more natural it becomes.

This is a great tool when eating out. Ask your waiter for a clean plate to be brought along with your meal. Your first plate becomes your serving dish and the clean one is your dining plate. This puts you in charge of how much food you think will satisfy you.

Remember, the people in the kitchen have to serve the same amount to everyone. No one knows how much food is right for you but *you.*

These tools will help you leave your meals feeling refreshed . . . and you just might be surprised how little it takes to truly satisfy when you're listening mindfully. Carry these good tools around with you and use them regularly. Pick one and master it. The skill of Mindful Eating is like any other skill—the more you practice the better you get at it and the more natural it becomes.

Not only do these tools help us enjoy our eating experiences more, they also help us stop eating when we are "just right" satisfied. This means we will be leaving food on our plates now. We no longer have to clean the plate. If this thought leaves you sad or uncomfortable, please know that this is perfectly normal. In the next chapter we will look closely at how to handle this.

Chapter 12

GRIEVING THE LOSS OF EXCESS AND CELEBRATING CHANGE

This Is Some of Your Most Important Work

*M*y former pastor, Dr. Doug Varnado, once captured my attention with this zinger statement: "When we tolerate overindulgence, we become dull." Why did these words resonate with me? Because I am very familiar with that deadening dullness.

Each of us is built to be fully alive, and our core knows it very well. We have deep longings and desires—far above pleasure. This conversation comes up all the time in workshop. It's not just being overweight or preoccupied that bothers us—it's what we know we're missing.

Certainly part of this great life is experiencing pleasure. But there are different kinds of pleasure. There are pleasures that enliven and there are pleasures that numb. There are pleasures that make us more ourselves and pleasures that make us less. When we continue to deaden ourselves with food—we are hiding part of our true selves.

Have you ever noticed after you've overeaten how hard it is to be fully available to yourself or others? I remember as a young mom feeling sad when I overate and then was groggy and regretful and not fully present with my children who I loved so much more than food.

Be encouraged! As you do the noble work of refusing the numbing plea-sure of overindulgence, you are freeing up and living out more and more of your true and genuine self.

To walk in this freedom we have to make some changes, don't we? Does the thought of waiting to eat when you're hungry, leaving food behind, not driving through the drive-thru whenever you think of it, stopping at "rea-sonable," dropping out of the Clean Plate Club, and being satisfied with less make you feel a little sad? If so, this is perfectly normal.

When we begin this journey of change, it's often true that there is sadness or grieving when a good meal is over, when we realize we've had enough before it's all gone or we see something yummy but know we're not hungry yet.

This grieving makes sense because overeating has meant something to us. And let's be honest, overdoing it feels really good while it's happening. I often hear people say that they have to have something sweet, and then something salty to balance it, and then something sweet . . . and then salty and on and on. This will never end if we don't understand and acknowledge our appetite for good taste is never going to be satisfied. Our appetite for pleasure is never fully or finally quenched. It will always return. Knowing this and expecting it is helpful. We *will* get hungry again. We *will* get to eat something yummy again. We don't have to eat it all now.

Liberated eating is the best choice we have for the most pleasure. This is big. Think it through. Stopping at satisfied gives you the pleasure of living in a healthy body and mind—*and* permission gives you the tastes you desire. But none of us—not even thin people—can eat *all* we want *anytime* we want, disregarding our body's needs and cries for moderation. This is an *Immovable*. And this may take some grieving.

We are going to face some sadness, but we can summon our courage and work through it.

There is great freedom on the other side!

You know how this sadness thing works; it's a catch-22. If you overeat, you feel the familiar heavy sadness of regret. If you leave food behind, you feel sad about not eating it.

In the beginning, you are going to be sad either way.

But understand, these two sadnesses have very different ends.

For a while:

> *You will either be*
> **SAD WITH REGRET**
> *or you will be*
> **SAD WITH REWARD.**

Reward is better.

So expect to feel some sadness right now. Decide ahead of time to tolerate it. When you feel sad over leaving food behind, acknowledge it and—as strange as it may sound—celebrate it. You are changing things and that's something to get excited about! This sadness (it can also feel like anxiety, anger or disappointment) will lessen and eventually end as you develop your new relationship with food.

I remember experiencing some unexpected disappointment as food began to take its rightful place in my life—when it was no longer my greatest thrill. That's really what this is all about, isn't it? We are wrestling with what place food is going to have in our lives. Of course this will be very uncomfortable at times. Sometimes it will feel like you're losing an old familiar friend—a dysfunctional friend, but friend nonetheless. Eating to excess is quick, easy gratification, total pleasure and fun. It doesn't argue or demand anything. This work of change demands something of us. It will take longer and be tougher duty than eating a box of Cheez-Its.

As we wrestle with what we truly want, tolerate some sadness and begin to stop at satisfied more often—even when we don't want to—we're going to feel things start to shift toward freedom. When it gets tough remind yourself of what is true.

Inner Dialogue: Talk Yourself Through

- *I'm free to eat whenever I'm hungry.*

- *Food is available anytime.*

- *There are no more diets in my future.*

- *I am free to eat, and I am free not to eat.*

You are doing the important work of *falling out of love with overeating* and *falling in love with feeling great*.

Remember to celebrate every large and small change, every choice, and every thought that is new—even while grieving. Those of us who struggle with food tend to see every little thing we think we've done wrong, and we tend to miss the myriad new things we are changing.

This is good work you are doing! Every effort is taking you in the direction of improved health and ultimate freedom. You might keep a list close by and begin to record any and everything that is not like it used to be.

Have a funeral if you need to.

If the sadness of stopping at satisfied (which means abandoning excess as a way of life) is overwhelming it may be time for a funeral. Be creative. This is your journey and there is no right or wrong way of doing it. Putting some formality to our losses can be powerful.

You may want to have a ceremony: dig a deep hole and bury a Super Sized Real Deal Meal and dance on the grave, grind

> You are falling out of love with overeating and falling in love with feeling great.

a whole bag of M&Ms up in the garbage disposal without eating one while singing a victory song real loud, or you may need to lay down and cry for a while. Whatever it takes. You are turning loose of something that has meant something to you in order to get what you want more. Let yourself grieve it.

After a discussion of *Grieving and Celebration*, Angie, who's been on this journey about seven months, put it eloquently:

> *God/life/circumstances have really been putting something in my face lately. And that's my tendency toward self-indulgence.*
>
> *Going through workshop has dramatically changed my eating world— but I've been struggling with this very thing Cindy is talking about. I miss my pig-out sessions. It was definitely a wonderful pleasure to be driving home with a bag of my favorite fast food and a huge soda. I miss baking cupcakes and eating half the batter while waiting for a batch to bake.*
>
> *It was a sweet self-indulgent time of marvelous sensations. All my senses involved. Self-medicating—oh how my concerns disappeared when I was eating that glorious food. I loved it!*
>
> *So, yes, I have grieved. Although those pig-out sessions always ended with regret—boy did I enjoy them at first.*

Here's what I realize, though: I've not been focusing on the second point—the celebration. It is a celebration! It is a victory every time I make an intuitive choice. How much more fulfilling life is when I can enjoy delicious food and look forward to a good meal with a reasonable level of anticipation—instead of being consumed by my obsession.

Instead of food being what fills me—now something else is taking up my emotional spaces: life! I am now focusing more on the world outside of me. The world outside of food. The less I focus on me—the more I see other people and the more I want to give. I can celebrate this!

I really like this idea of letting it go. I might just throw myself on my bed and flail around, kick and yell as loud as I can, beat on the mattress and cry a while, because I definitely have been grieving. And I want to get it out and let it go. I'm about to be done with it.

I'm ready for life. For living and breathing and fresh air and moving more and eating intuitively. For the greater pleasure that comes from loving others . . . and, yes, from loving myself too. Oh the sweet joy. It's way better than a chocolate chip cookie. I promise you, it is.

Wow, this is doing the good work of change. This is falling out of love with overeating and falling in love with being fully alive.

WHAT HAPPENS BETWEEN HUNGER AND SATISFACTION? Part 1

Permission to Eat What Satisfies

We have looked closely at waiting on our true hunger and stopping when we're satisfied—but what takes place *between* these two important steps? Let's look at some practices that will make for an enjoyable and health-giving eating experience.

Keep in mind that at first the act of mindfulness will probably feel odd. You may feel hyper-conscious, as you did when first learning to ride a bike or drive a car. You may, at times, feel it is impossible to change your deep tendencies to eat quickly or on autopilot. Let me assure you that countless people, just like you and me, have felt this very same way. And they have marveled at the glory of the change once they got into their journey.

Here's Carol:

I am shocked! I simply never thought I would say this, but I am becoming the kind of person that used to annoy me. I occasionally forget to eat! Also, waiting for hunger is becoming so natural to me that I almost never think about it anymore. I just do it. It feels right. To be honest, I really didn't think this Liberated Eating thing would work for me because my eating was so out of whack. Now I don't want to eat when I'm not hungry. It is even becoming easy and natural to make healthy choices. And almost no more "crazy-eating" alone or in public. I eat like a normal person. I am proud of the patience I have developed, waiting for hunger and sitting when I am not sure. I love that I have found my "full" button again; it was lost for decades. The changes that have occurred inside this head, heart, soul, and body (including my stomach!) this past year have been amazing. I honestly feel like another person, especially psychologically. A lot of healing has been done. I wouldn't trade this journey and work for anything and would never want to go back. Being free from obsessing about food has to be one of the greatest things that has ever happened to me.

This kind of freedom is possible for each of us.

So, we're checking in to see if we're hungry and deciding how hungry we are. What next?

Eat What You Want

(Read this section slowly, this concept can rock your world . . .)

Go ahead—choose what you will enjoy eating. Does this seem too good to be true? Dangerous? Maybe even wicked?

This is the part of the liberated eating message that always raises the most eyebrows. We tend to think that if we have freedom we will abuse it. Experience and research bear out that when people eat according to their body's signals and eat what is satisfying to them, they do not overeat and they do eventually make nutritionally balanced choices.

Bess, who is now sixty pounds lighter, put it this way:

It took me a while after workshop to trust that anything in moderation is fine. Now if I want to eat something I have it. It is no longer the ordeal. I choose mostly healthy when hungry, stop eating when full and really enjoy food for the first time ever. My weight release journey continues simply because now food is not the focal point in my life. Food has been replaced by other great feelings of joy!

This story is echoed over and over again. Moving from rigid food rules to permission opens the door for an authentic, intuitive, livable relationship with food.

Listen to Dr. Tracy Tylka of Ohio State University. She and her team have studied Intuitive Eating for years.

There's this belief that if you give people unconditional permission to eat, they are going to binge and add on a lot of pounds. But that's not what we have found. It seems amazing, but it is true. If you listen to your body signals in determining what, when, and how much to eat, you are not going to binge and you're going to eat an appropriate amount of nutrient-dense foods.

Dr. Tylka's extensive studies found that those who followed intuitive eating principles had a lower Body Mass Index, were less influenced by our culture's obsession with thinness and were generally more optimistic than those who did not.[5]

Relaxed, instinctive eaters routinely eat what they really want to eat. They fix or order what they want—not what they think they *should* eat. They don't feel guilty or noble about their choices. They enjoy their food and often leave a lot behind. How are they able to do this? Because they aren't choosing from "should." Choosing what they want for lunch is not a moral issue. They're choosing from a place of honesty and freedom. As Dr. May says in her good book *Eat What You Love, Love What You Eat*, "When guilt is no longer a factor, common sense prevails."

Satisfaction is not just for your body. Your mind needs to be happy about eating too. When we eat foods that aren't pleasant to us— foods we think we "should" be eating—our body may be fed but our mind is not satisfied. This makes it probable that we will continue to graze until we are satisfied. There seems to be no way around it—we must allow ourselves to eat foods we enjoy!

> Freedom is not the absence of self-control. It is the ability to train our desires for good; the privilege to rightly order our loves and lives.

Certainly all foods are not the same nutritionally, and intuitive eaters know this. They make choices that are healthful with room for some "fun foods" that don't bring much nutrition to the table. These fun foods are enjoyed without guilt but end up being a small part of their overall menu.

This happens because intuitive eaters are being *intuitive*. Intuition tells us that we want to keep our body working at peak performance, which demands enough nutritious fuel to do so. Intuitive eaters know more than a few bites of a very rich dessert will leave them wanting a nap. They will choose foods that taste good and make them feel energized for the next part of the day.

If you really want a certain food but think you *should not* have it, you will probably continue wanting it—giving that food more power over you than it ever needed to have. In this situation we often end up eating it anyway—and probably overeating it.

What's a person to do? *Begin to live in a new reality*—one that makes sense. Remember, our goal is to thrive. Filter everything through this high mission.

 Core Belief

EAT WHAT YOU [AND YOUR BODY] WANT

I give myself permission to eat what I want. There are no illegal foods. Since I want to feel refreshed after I eat, I choose a variety of foods that will satisfy my taste buds and energize my whole body.

A Whole New Question for a Whole New Health, Satisfaction and Freedom

As restrictive eaters we've been asking the wrong question. We've been asking, "What should I eat?" which also implies, "What shouldn't I eat?" This makes the decision process a moral issue when it is not. It's very difficult to make an honest or satisfying decision when you think you will be either a good or bad person depending on what you choose to eat.

Not a helpful question:
"What should I eat?"

A very helpful question:
"What's going to make me feel great—now and later?"

As liberated eaters we want to be well and to feel satisfied with our eating experience. When we're living this way we can look at the choices available and ask, "What's going to make me feel good—both now *and* later on today?" We are addressing both pleasure and health.

We are taking the whole picture into account: What will taste best to me right now? What will sit well in my stomach right now? What will give me good energy for the next four or five hours?

At first it may not be easy to make a pure decision if you've been choosing from the diet perspective for many years. You will get good at it with practice. Relax and remind yourself of what is true.

Inner Dialogue: Talk Yourself Through

- *I can choose without anxiety because I'm eating when my body needs fuel (I've checked in and I'm hungry). I'm doing the wise thing at the best time.*

- *I'm free to choose what I want because there are no illegal foods now.*

- *Since I want to feel great all day, I'm going to choose what will satisfy my taste buds, my mind, and my energy/health needs.*

- *I can afford to stop when I feel my body is satisfied, no matter how much food is left, because I can always eat again when I'm hungry.*

Not long ago Renee explained how great this permission felt to her.

When the new peanut butter Snickers came out I just had to try it. Normally I would have obsessed over it and felt guilty and sneaky about going into a store and buying a candy bar—almost criminal! I would have tried to talk myself out of it—then I would have bought more than one and eaten them all in the parking lot thinking that I would never eat them again after this—so I better get my fill.

With the freedom of permission in my mind, it was a completely different experience. While I was doing my regular shopping I bought the candy bar just like a normal person [You are, Renee!], put it in the pantry when I got home, and waited for true hungry. When I got hungry for lunch, I put the Snickers on a plate, cut it into pieces with a knife, looked at it, smelled it, savored it, and enjoyed it thoroughly. I had milk with it and some turkey and cheese for dessert. It was a wonderful lunch. There was no guilt! I felt peaceful and very satisfied.

It is true that we may gravitate toward the formerly "illegal" foods when we first begin this journey, but this will balance out.

We're a lot like a prisoner of war who's been shut up in a tiny, dark cell for years. When he is finally free, he may sleep outside under the stars for a while just to prove to himself that he is *truly* free, but he will eventually sleep in a bed like the rest of us. Give yourself a little time to freely exercise your newfound liberty and you will begin to feel yourself relax.

Here are some things to keep in mind about permission:

Don't let any foods stay on the "illegal" list. Coming to believe that you can have *any* food *any* time is part of letting food become neutral—which is an important part of reclaiming the intuitive eater in you. *[Of course, the ultimate goal is to be well so it is understood that permission to eat anything does not mean disregarding medical issues, energy needs, allergies, etc.]*

We won't gain weight when we're eating between hunger and satisfaction. We have never gained weight because of *what* we've eaten. Thin people eat cake on occasion. We have gained weight because of *how much* of it we've eaten and because we've eaten when we weren't hungry.

Be brave, and embrace variety! Variety is a big part of feeling satisfied for most people. Research shows that disordered eaters often eat the same ten to fifteen things over and over again.

Over time it takes more and more of these foods to give the same satisfaction smaller amounts used to give. Most intuitive eaters tend to eat smaller amounts of more variety.

You can control yourself with particularly tempting food. Certain foods can feel especially powerful over us. Maybe there is a memory attached to that food, which makes you feel especially good when you eat it.

Cathy and her sister grew up with an angry, volatile, alcoholic father. Often when he left the house for evening shift, their mother tried to sooth their hurt with food, saying, "Come on, girls. Let's have some fun! Let's get in the kitchen and bake something wonderful." Is it any wonder that sweet treats triggered a deep emotional response in Cathy's heart?

One way to handle an "irresistible food" is to have a lot of that food around. This idea may sound dangerous at first, but consider this: What would happen if you could have this irresistible food for breakfast, lunch, and dinner—for days or even weeks? This approach will eventually take that food off the pedestal and put it down on neutral ground with all other foods. I have done this with donuts, which I felt were "the nectar of the gods" for years—so forbidden, so "fattening," so heavenly that I, a mere mortal, shouldn't even look on them. Of course, this led to regular donut binges, weight gain, and regret.

> A few days or weeks of the same thing, no matter how great it is, will take the "special" right off.

Remember—if we use this process, we are still honoring hunger and satisfaction. This is our firm foundation. This approach is not an excuse to harm ourselves by overeating.

A few days or weeks of the same thing, no matter how great it is, will take the "special" right off. You may have to go through this process again later if it's particularly strong, but you will eventually come to believe that you really can eat anything you want when you're hungry—which means that "forbidden" foods will have lost their false power over you. A good, cold, juicy pear and chocolate pudding will be the same in emotional weight.

Important: To keep blood sugar normal, it's a good idea to have some protein with your meal. Since I am hypoglycemic I had some tuna, turkey, nuts, beans or an egg as an appetizer and then ate my donut. Otherwise I would have felt weak and shaky.

Here's what Laura said about her experience with normalizing her love/hate relationship with chocolate.

For as long as I can remember I have eaten chocolate when I have been in pain. The more I ate, the more I wanted it. I told myself I would not buy more once it was all gone, so I would eat all that I had . . . but then I'd buy more. In workshop, Cindy suggested the option of buying lots of chocolate and keeping it around my house. I was very fearful of this idea. I decided to try it since I didn't know what else to do. I remember being in the grocery store and making the decision not to hide what I was doing but rather to embrace it. I bought many bags of chocolate as well as large bars of all sorts. I brought it all home and put some of it in a candy jar where I could see it. I let my family and friends know what I was doing. Initially I ate quite a bit, but not more than I had when I was bingeing on it daily. Within a few days, I was not thinking about it and I had several bags left in my kitchen. I can say that I have not binged on chocolate again since that time. I know I can have it whenever I want to.

Let your own wisdom guide you. This approach is not for everyone in every situation. For me there are some foods, like homemade pies, that are special to me and I want them to remain special. They sing from a place in my childhood and connect me with my fore-mothers. I enjoy baking one when we have company, knowing we can enjoy it together and that there will not be much left—maybe just a slice for breakfast the next day. I don't keep them around my home regularly. Again, let your own wisdom prevail for you.

So, we have left diet foods behind and have joined the ranks of "normal" eaters and are free to choose food we really do want to eat. Now what?

Chapter 14

WHAT HAPPENS BETWEEN HUNGER AND SATISFACTION? Part 2

Show Up, Slow Down & Savor, Think Like a Connoisseur, Be Mindful of Amounts and Posture

*J*magine that you have checked in and found that you are physically hungry and now you have food sitting before you that "hits the spot." Let's discover how to enjoy this meal to its full satisfaction and your best health.

Show Up

Let your mind show up before your mouth starts eating. Being connected with your eating experience gives you more of everything you love—more taste, more enjoyment, more fun, more gratitude, more energy, more contentment, more satisfaction.

In our frenetic culture, it's easy to gulp down a meal and barely remember it. We eat while driving, walking around, checking e-mails, and watching TV. We think about food all day long except while we're eating it! Figure that one out.

Eating mindfully is *deliberate*. The root word of deliberate is *liberate*, which is exactly what we're after. We are becoming liberated. Our main job now is to be present during our eating experience—to be truly connected. When we eat this way, *we remember it* and then we don't feel like prowling around for food all day. We can get on with life.

After this lesson, Hudson came into workshop the following week with the perfect illustration.

One day around lunch time he was working at his computer when he called to his wife in another room, "Hey, Patty, where's my tuna sub?" There was a little pause and she said, "Look in the trash." Sure enough there was the bag, the wrapper, and no tuna sub. He had eaten an entire sandwich and had no recollection of it. None. He had eaten every bite—but had no satisfaction from it. He wanted to eat another one because the first one just hadn't registered.

Remember to let your mind *show up* before your mouth starts eating. It's so much easier to be mindful when your mind is there to help you.

So how do we show up? You have to set the stage for remembering your eating experience. As you read the ideas below, consider them time-proven guidelines—not rules—to help you figure out what will work for you. This is not pass/fail. This is about discovery and change.

 Setting the Stage for Mindfulness

- **Sit down to eat.** It's preferable to do so at a table meant for dining. This sets your eating time apart from the rest of your day. You might even put a napkin in your lap. (If you sit a lot you might wish to stand at a tall table. We can be mindful while standing as well.)
- **Use a plate.** Using a plate brings awareness. It's an intentional act that marks the moment for eating. Getting a small plate for your snack rather than eating from a bag or putting your take-out meal on a real plate helps you be mindful.
- **Reframe mealtime.** Think of this moment in your day as a refreshing break, as a moment that deserves time and attention. Do your best to give each meal about twenty minutes. Put away the phone, computer, TV, work, etc. This can feel uncomfortable

or irritating at first. The cool thing is that after you get through the initial awkwardness, you will treasure the refreshing experience deeply.

 ### *Arrive Before the First Bite*

The tools below will keep you from plopping down and immediately flying in with the fork in high gear and rushing right through the meal. There are many ways to do this and you'll find your favorites. This will only take a few seconds after some practice.

- **Breathe.** Take a few deep breaths. You might like to close your eyes. Let your core relax and tension melt away.
- **Become aware of being in your body.** This may sound a little goofy, but we can be so distracted that we really are not aware of our body. Notice your weight sitting in the seat, your feet on the floor, and your spine against the chair. Connect with your body.
- **Use your senses.** Notice your immediate surroundings. Identify one smell, two sounds, and three objects.
- **Focus on the food in front of you.** What do you smell first? What textures and colors are most interesting? What part looks most appetizing to you?
- **Be wowed!** Look at your food and be amazed. Trace one food all the way back to its origin in your mind. Think of all the people and energy it took to get this food to a plate. Those beans in that burrito used to be out in a sunny field!
- **Feel Grateful.** Say grace. Gratitude is a great connector.

As you get more and more mindful experiences under your belt, notice how you feel when you return to the day after this twenty-minute mini-vacation. This intentional investment in a pleasant eating experience is going to bring a new quality to your whole day—and that belt will get looser too.

Treat Yourself

Dare to *fully* enjoy one meal a day. Start with one. Wait for true hunger, pick what will satisfy, make yourself comfortable, create a pleasant dining space, allow no distractions, take a deep breath, set your inner pace to "relaxed," maybe put on your favorite music. Simply enjoy your food, your own company, or the company of others. Notice how you feel before, during, and after the meal. Try this for a few weeks and check your energy and satisfaction factor.

Slow Down and Savor

We instinctively slow down and savor non-food things that we enjoy. We linger over conversation with a friend, leaning in to drink every good thing from the moment. We long for time to stand still when we happen upon a stunning sunset. We never say, "This movie is so good, let's fast forward!" or "Let's hurry through this awesome vacation!" We want good things to last.

So why do we eat quickly?

This is a very good question. Next time you find yourself hurrying through a meal . . . stop . . . and ask yourself *why?* Really. "Why am I eating so quickly?" It may take some thought to get to the real answer, but it will be invaluable insight. Perhaps you don't like the food or you feel obligated to eat it, or you are pushed for time. Maybe you're anxious or uncomfortable. Maybe it's a habit or you let yourself get too hungry. Whatever the reason or reasons, once you identify them you are halfway home to changing things!

Speed is a big deal when it comes to your health, so let's look at why it is so important to change:

- When we eat quickly, we usually race right past "full" and don't even know it. About twenty minutes after the meal we realize we're uncomfortable and groggy.
- The faster we eat the less the eating experience registers, leaving us unsatisfied and still wanting more even though the belly is full.
- The faster we eat the more we eat. Eating fast leads to weight gain.
- Our appetite adapts to larger and larger amounts of food as we race through mindlessly. It takes more and more food, over time, to get the same thrill less used to provide.

Dr. Wansink's very interesting book *Mindless Eating* (a great one to add to your wellness library), points us to some very telling information[6] concerning our eating pace.

Why do we stop eating a meal? When I ask this in workshop, I always hear from some clever soul, "Because the food is gone." You would think that we stop when full. Turns out it's more complicated than that. Scientists think it's a combination of things:

1. ***How much we chew.*** Our body kind of has a "chew quota." It has to chew enough to know it's been fed. Guess that's why sometimes a smoothie leaves me wanting a little something else.

2. ***How much we taste.*** We have a "taste quota" too. We miss a lot of good taste when we gulp down big bites in a hurry.

3. ***How much we connect with the food.*** Our mind and body want to know they have eaten. Connecting is really hard to do while speeding down the road, or checking Facebook, or watching TV. Our mind is just not able to connect at a satisfying level.

4. ***How much we swallow.*** We have a "swallow quota" as well. If we eat that piece of pizza in five big bites, we don't get many swallows. If we take reasonable bites and chew well we have more swallowing satisfaction.

5. ***How long we have been eating.*** Your stomach and hypothalamus need time to sort things out. They can't be rushed. They need about twenty minutes to chat about being well-fueled.

These things add up to this: *Eating quickly works against your health.*

Slowing Down Means Buying New Pants

Dr. Wansink had another bit of very fascinating information that shines the light on the importance of eating at a reasonable pace. Research shows that consistently eating slowly leads us to be satisfied with 70 calories of fuel *less* per meal. This is theoretically 210 calories less daily (if you happen to eat three meals per day) which adds up to releasing twenty-one pounds in a year. Sounds like something worth working on!

Core Belief

ENJOY EACH BITE

I enjoy my food. I sit down to eat, making sure I am fully present.
I have a relaxed posture, take reasonably sized bites and chew
slowly—savoring the good gift of food.

For optimal digestion, your stomach likes to receive its meals almost lique-
fied. This is why we have those big, grinding molars. The suggested chews
for most effective digestion are around twenty-five to thirty chews per bite.
Taking medium sized bites—not large ones—is also key to good digestion.

It's an eye opening experience to begin to be more mindful of bite size
and chewing. As we experiment with this in workshop, I am always surprised
how many people are highly affected by this. It is the key to some people
truly enjoying their food on a whole new level. Chewing is a big deal.

One of my nurse friends told me that when she feeds a comatose patient
through a feeding tube directly into the stomach, even though the food
never enters their mouth, the patient will often begin to chew in their sleep.
(Why does this make me want to cry a little?) Chewing, nourishment, and
digestion are intricately connected and intuitive for us.

Warning: Chain Chewing Is Dangerous for Your Health

Chain chewing is the process of putting another bite in your mouth before
the last one is swallowed. It's continually putting new food on top of half-
chewed food. This popular technique makes it impossible to distinguish one
bite from the next and leads to overeating, under-chewing and missing a lot
of pleasure.

Try this experiment next time you're eating. Put a bite in your mouth,
then *put your fork down* and concentrate on that one bite. Enjoy that bite
fully, paying attention to the flavors, temperature, textures. Keep up your
mindfulness as you chew and swallow, noticing the after-tastes when the
food is gone. One bite can be an amazing experience!

Take a drink and get ready for the next bite. While you're chewing the next bite, load your fork and hold it in eyesight. Notice the difference in your connection with the first bite and the second.

You can't concentrate on the bite you're chewing because your mind is focused on loading the fork and the bite that's coming next. This is how the brain works—it looks ahead unless we consciously slow it down and tell it what to concentrate on.

So you can see the crazy thing that happens when we always have the next bite waiting. We miss the bite in our mouth and it's the only one we can enjoy.

 Tools for Relaxing Your Eating Pace

Chain chewing means you never actually fully experience the bite in your mouth, which is where the party happens! These tools (again, not rules) can help you find your relaxed eating pace:

- Put your fork or food down between bites.
- Take a drink of water between bites.
- Use chop sticks or children's utensils.
- Eat with your non-dominant hand.
- Set a timer for twenty minutes and enjoy your meal slowly until it goes off. This can be fun for family meals and brings awareness to everyone.
- Two-Minute Mid-Meal Pause (from chapter 11) is a great tool for resetting the pace halfway through your meal.
- Play musical chairs. Each meal sit in a different place at the table so you're more aware of where you are and less on auto-pilot.

One more important point here: Make sure you *eat before you're famished!* It is so hard to eat at a relaxed pace if you are very hungry, especially for those of us with dieting in our recent past. The memory of deprivation can still be working in us to cause some desperation when extreme hunger is felt.

Snacks can help, so do yourself a favor and have some in your car or purse in case you find yourself in a place where true hunger hits and you don't have a meal close by. Raw almonds are a good choice for me because they keep a long time and they aren't *so, so* good that I have to work very hard to resist eating them just for fun. I have permission to eat anything—but I don't keep cookies under the driver's seat.

 Thinking Like a Connoisseur

Who enjoys food more than a connoisseur? Every bite is intentionally savored—every sense employed. Nothing is rushed. Every little detail is scrutinized for quality and is fully appreciated. Now I'm not suggesting we become irritatingly picky, but I am suggesting that going into a food situation with the mindset of a connoisseur will benefit us in many ways.

A connoisseur has an open, fully engaged, vigorous attitude toward food—not one of shame or fear. A connoisseur eats with ease in public—no shame, no hiding.

The benefits of thinking like a connoisseur are exactly what we're looking for—*intentional liberated mindfulness.*

A connoisseur will eat the best food, enjoy it more than anyone else, and not waste time on mediocre food. They know that if the first bite isn't great, it won't get any better.

What would happen if you fully tasted everything you ate? Here's a fun experiment[7] that will help you experience one fully tasted bite:

TASTING AT CONNOISSEUR LEVEL

1. Choose a bite carefully. Just the right bite. Just the right size, maybe smaller than usual so you can taste every bit.

2. Before you take the bite, smell the food and enjoy the aromas.

3. Look at the food. Become fully aware of every detail.

4. During the bite, shut out all other stimuli. If it helps, close your eyes for a few seconds. Concentrate on this one bite—the taste, the texture, the temperature, the individual flavors. As much as possible, engage all five senses.

5. Continue to chew until this one bite is thoroughly chewed.

6. Swallow and wait. Do not automatically grab another bite. Notice any aftertastes and savor them.

At first, devote *one* bite per meal to tasting fully. Then, go to *two* bites for some meals, and then *three*. Work up to occasionally eating an entire meal in this way.

Dieting hasn't just separated us from our intuition; it has damaged our discernment and pure appreciation for good and real food. We

> We can enjoy many delicious foods in this life and keep our good health when we realize that quantity is not what makes it a pleasure.

often feel that we don't deserve good food, believing that *real food* is for skinny people. We have often settled for mediocre food (or worse) and less-than-satisfying eating experiences—the whole time trying to convince ourselves that this frozen, no-fat, no-taste chicken dinner is really yummy. It's time to take back our enjoyment, our judgment, and our taste buds!

I used to think that I was absolutely wicked if I ate real cheese. Cheese is a BIG DIET NO-NO. There was the plastic diet variety of course—but real cheese was just out of the question. Now I enjoy every new cheese I can find. I have become a bit of a cheese adventurer. The deli lady at the grocery store points me to new ones because she knows I'll be as excited as she is.

We can see our way clear to many wonderful eating experiences once we understand that it is never the food that "makes us fat." It's how much of it we eat and eating when we aren't hungry that gets us in trouble.

I once met a French pastry chef who was quite thin. She ate a few perfect bites of pastry every day. They were little treasures to her, and she knew that one bite treasured was much better than three pastries gobbled.

We can enjoy many delicious foods in this life *and* keep our good health when we realize that *quantity* is not what makes it a pleasure.

Practice saying these statements:

- Cheese is not fattening.
- Whipped cream is not fattening.
- Chocolate is not fattening.
- Food is not fattening.
- Enjoying food is not fattening.

And these:

- Eating when I'm not hungry is fattening.[8]
- Eating past satisfied is fattening.

- Eating for the sake of *quantity* is fattening.
- Eating quickly is fattening.
- Eating mindlessly is fattening.

Start letting yourself become comfortable with the truth that you can live well with food. You are living in a whole new reality now—one that makes sense. Thinking like a connoisseur will help. And besides, it's fun.

Become Mindful of Serving Sizes

If we lived in our great grandparents' time we would not be having this discussion.

If Maw Maw and Pop got a hankerin' for crispy fried chicken, they had to catch it, kill it, scald it, pluck it, cut it, flour it, and fry it—not to mention chop the wood and build the fire. By the time they got it to the table they had already used more fuel than they were about to eat. In a matter of minutes we can get to the drive-thru window, hand over the plastic, and drive away with a bucket of the stuff, a gallon of tea, and three sides.

Being aware of serving size and packaging is more important now than it has ever been because our food is always available in cheap, super-tasty abundance.

Serving sizes have changed in our lifetime. Plates are now the size of platters. Pizzas are the size of small trampolines. One restaurant portion can often feed three or four people. I read recently that the average restaurant meal is between 1,000 and 1,500 calories of fuel now. Most people's bodies don't want or need more than around 500 to 600 at a time (excluding the very active). Our food is served in WHOPPER portions. And food itself has changed as well—more on that later.

The problem is this: We tend to think we're done when we've finished "one portion," which appears to be whatever is set before us.

As very young children we would *not* do this. We stopped eating when our little tummy said to. But after we heard for the millionth time "Clean your plate" and "Eat your vegetables before you can have dessert" and "Just eat five more bites," the intuitiveness was wrung right out of us.

I'm sure most of this was well-meaning—perhaps a leftover backlash from the Great Depression or a desire for us to get enough nutrients—but now we have some damage control to do.

Think about this:

If we usually eat what is put before us, and we are continually over-served, what is inevitable?

We are going to get sicker and sicker.

It's time for some serious reframing when it comes to eating at a restaurant or zipping through a drive-thru. The cooks do not know you. They serve the same portion size to everyone. They don't know how hungry you are, how tall you are, how old you are, or how active you've been today.

No one but you knows how hungry you are. No one but you knows what you would like to eat. No one but you knows when you are pleasantly satisfied. You are the expert on YOU. Remember that.

The same principle applies to snack foods. What would happen if you opened a Milky Way, savored three bites, and . . . put the rest away? Who says that whole bar is what you want? Who knows that but you? We often automatically eat to the end of whatever is packaged without thinking about it. *Until now!* Do not let anyone or anything tell you how much you would like to eat. They simply cannot know.

When we become mindful of this, we have just become those people who eat what they want but don't overeat. Understand the magnitude of this. A breakthrough in this area is life changing.

How Can I Waste This Perfectly Good Food?

So you might be thinking this is all well and good but throwing away two-thirds of a meal or a candy bar when you just paid good money for it is sticking in your craw.

I get this. This is a conversation that comes up over and over again.

Of course it is a good thing to be wise with our hard-earned money. Couple that with the feeling of desperation about food left over from our dieting days and we have a problem with leaving food behind. But that leads to a much more serious problem—we are eating stuff that's slowly killing us and thinking that we're saving money.

Earth to us: This is ludicrous!

Let's think this through. Whatever we spend on a meal is a sunk cost. If you pay twelve dollars for dinner, you spend twelve dollars whether you eat it all or eat two bites. If you eat past full, you hurt your stomach, you upset your blood sugar level, you tax your digestion, you feel heavy and tired, and you store the extra fuel as fat, which does more harm than just making your pants tight. On top of all that, you probably feel guilty too. This is not a deal.

You can bring food home. You can leave it right there and let someone else clear the table. You can split a meal with someone else. There are many options here, but one thing is clear: *You never save money when you overeat.*

Look at the definition of the word *waste*—to use or expend to no purpose; to use without adequate return; useless consumption.

This is very interesting—we tend to think we're wasting food or money by leaving food on our plate when actually we are wasting the food and the money when the eating is not used for its intended purpose. When we hit satisfied, the money is well spent and the purpose of fueling is accomplished. The food eaten after that has no true purpose. It is wasted.

Here is another thought that can appeal to our rational selves: Medical bills as a result of being overweight are much greater than any savings we imagine come from cleaning our plate. If you're young, this may not hit home yet, but just ask friends over sixty and they will explain. Get well and get well now. Eating the other half of a $7 sub when your body doesn't want it does not save you $3.50. It costs you *a lot more.*

Enjoy that sub just the way you like it. When your very smart stomach says quit, stop and celebrate the money and health you've just saved. *Reprogram* your mind on this very important point.

Posture: The Outside Can Affect the Inside . . . and Visa Versa

Now we know to show up, slow down and savor, chew reasonably-sized bites well, think like a connoisseur, and be mindful of serving sizes. Let's look at one last thing.

How we sit (or not) at the table—our posture toward the food and the moment—can have an effect on everything else we've discussed. I'm not talking about the kind of posture your health teacher encouraged—just sitting up straight, although that probably wouldn't hurt. I'm talking about taking a relaxed and engaged posture that can start the whole eating experience off mindfully.

This may sound like an odd assignment, but begin to notice people's posture as they eat. Some are relaxed and engaged, some tense and hurried. Some seem concerned that their food might be taken from them while others are focused on their phones and are a million miles from their eating experience. Some lean far back away from the table and others bend down over their food so the fork has a short trip . . . it's fascinating.

Begin to notice your own posture as well. Remember to be the curious observer, not the critical judge. As a scientist neutrally observes, make your observations without judgment or assumption.

What is your relationship/posture toward your plate, fork, food, table, and company? Is it a relaxed, engaged posture or a frantic attack posture? Do you seem calm and open to refreshment or preoccupied and unable to experience the true pleasure of a meal? If our posture is an outward indication of an inward attitude, what would you say yours is? Some of us are programmed to rush through certain meals because of past schedules. Are you more relaxed and engaged at certain meals than others?

Be intentional about posture. We can choose to sit at the table in a way that opens us up to being blessed, in a way that honors our health, the meal, the one who prepared it, the company we share, and this moment in the day. Begin to experiment with the posture that serves you well. Only you will know.

The relaxing practice of mindfulness helps us switch our focus from the food to the dining experience. As dieters we have been food-focused and have often missed the lovely experience of dining—until now.

Remember that food is a good gift—not the enemy. It would certainly be easy for us to think that food is the enemy after trying to control it for years. We've tried to hold it at bay—fighting valiantly with our paltry diet weapons only to end up right back where we started. Food was never the problem, and as long as we believe *food* causes us to overeat we are handicapped. That myth gives food power it really does not have.

As we become more and more mindful and intuitive, we also become more and more empowered to live with the health and weight we desire. You don't have to do all these things perfectly, but as you practice you will see the old ineffective ways drop by the wayside and the new, strong, health-giving ways take root and grow. Your pants will get looser and your mind will be freer.

Get fierce about this journey! Wake up in the morning and remind yourself where you're headed. Go to bed at night with life-giving truths on your mind. Keep an inspiring wellness book by the bed, make some note cards with your favorite thoughts on them or keep a journal for you journaling types—whatever keeps you supported, *do it*. Change it when it gets dull. Keep your wellness vision polished up and in focus. Remember how badly you want this—and that you certainly can have it.

We've looked closely at how we can find our path to freedom with the good gift of food. Now let's look at what might drive us to eat when we aren't hungry and how to navigate it.

PART III

The Emotional Side of Things

Changing the Conversation in Your Head and Heart

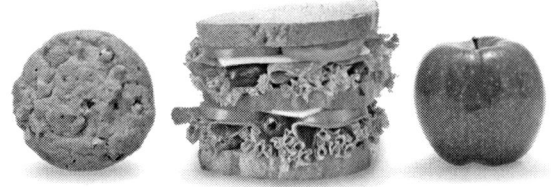

Chapter 15

RECOGNIZING WHAT'S DRIVING YOU TO EAT

Internal, External and Emotional Cues

*N*ow that we've taken a good look at what it takes to live well with food behaviorally (the *how*)—let's look more closely at what's going on in our heads and hearts (the *why*). Our behaviors are intrinsically connected to what's going on in there.

It can feel as though there are a million reasons to eat, but when we boil it all down there are basically only three. It helps to know this so we can determine which of these reasons is driving us to eat:

- Internal cues (physical hunger—we need fuel)
- External cues (smell popcorn, see ad for chewy brownies)
- Emotional cues (feel stressed, bored, happy, angry, etc.)

When we're aware of the reasons we want to eat, we can respond from a place of understanding. We can drive *it* instead of it driving us!

Internal Cues

We already know about this first desire to eat. True, physical hunger is an internal cue that is *connected* to the real needs of your body. It works for you and your health. This is, inarguably, the only way to live peacefully and healthfully with food. The best thing is that it is *by far* the most glorious way to eat—food tastes better and satisfies more completely when we eat because our body needs fuel. We can always trust that we're eating at the right time when we're physically hungry.

External Cues

These cues are from the outside world. We could think of external cues as being in one of these three categories:

- advertisements, commercials, marketing
- food that shows up unexpectedly (your neighbor brings over half her son's birthday cake because she doesn't want it in her house)
- food you expected to show up and, sure enough, it did (every time you visit your grandmom she has Rice Krispies treats)

All three of these are disconnected from the real needs of your body. When eating in response to an external cue, you can work *against* yourself, your goals and your health.

Think about all the things around you that "remind" you to eat when you're *not* hungry. External cues are everywhere! Pizza advertisements you can practically smell, savory cheeseburgers you can get on every corner without ever leaving your car, huge billboards of cold, refreshing soft drinks, warm cookies in hotel lobbies, your own pantry and freezer full of ready-to-eat goodies, candy dishes brimming, hot donuts in the break room. You cannot go *anywhere* that food is not offered!

No other generation in all of human history has had to contend with this—except for some French kings who died of gout if they didn't lose their heads first. We really are in a unique position, and since it's probably not going to change, we have to learn how to respond reasonably in our unreasonable situation. And we can.

> Stop watching. Stop listening. Stop drooling. Take your life back! Don't let anyone tell you what to crave.

One thing each of us must do is make a personal decision about what place advertising is going to have in our lives. This is serious. People are sitting around a table right now figuring out how to make you want what you aren't even thinking about yet. Ten billion dollars is spent each year advertising food and beverages to children and youth alone.[9] Just food and beverages. Just to children and youth.

Do advertisements affect you? Do you get a particular food on your mind and then feel deprived if you don't have it? Advertising is effective—corporations would not spend billions if it weren't. We must put some supports in place so we reach our goal of optimal health instead of helping advertisers reach their goal of optimal wealth.

There is one very effective solution. Stop watching. Stop listening. Stop drooling. Stop being bewitched and beguiled. Mute, unhook, cancel subscriptions. Take your life back! Don't let anyone tell you what to crave—especially someone who is not the least bit interested in your health. You have to get fierce about this. I haven't watched a commercial in years (in my own home) and I don't receive magazines full of them. I promise you that after the initial withdrawal, you will be infinitely more peaceful and free.

You are responsible for the messages you allow into our life. You are responsible for the stewardship of your mind and body. No one can do this for you.

Let's look at other external cues. Popcorn at the theatre, abundant holiday goodies, monthly birthday parties, cinnamon rolls at morning meetings, cookies in cookie jars . . . it's endless.

Whenever these situations arise, and they will regularly, we can depend on our mindfulness and intuition to lead us through. We can go anywhere with any kind of food and walk away satisfied—this is a powerful thing to realize and remember. We are not asking ourselves not to eat certain foods. We're just asking ourselves not to overeat.

 Standing Firm in the Face of External Cues

Here are some powerful "thought resources" you can rely on to help you stand firm when faced with external pressures to eat. Have them ready when needed. It won't be long.

> *Stop. Breathe. Recognize.* Step away from the food and take a few deep breaths before you do anything. Breathing actually helps you clear your mind and not automatically default to old patterns. As you breathe, remind yourself that you're in charge.
>
> Recognize this situation as one in which you could be sidetracked, but do not have to be. You might say to yourself, "Just

because food appears, this does not mean I or my goals have to be side-tracked. It's just food. It's everywhere! I can get this anytime I want it." Remember that you can accomplish what you want to accomplish in spite of obstacles. You've got this. This food is not illegal. It has no power over you. You can have it. You can choose *not* to have it.

Every time you walk away, you will be more and more confident and able to do it again. You will see that it doesn't hurt, that it feels great in fact! I just received this e-mail: "I went somewhere this morning where they had cinnamon rolls. I had already had breakfast and was not even tempted . . . I got a bottle of water . . . Yeah!!! I am eating a peach as I hit send." Bravo! You can hear the thrill of victory.

Remember what you REALLY, REALLY want. Have your wellness vision vivid and ever ready. You—feeling strong, energetic and light in your mind and body—walking down the beach at sunset, hiking a mountain trail, dancing, your doctor telling you to stop your meds because your numbers are so good.

Remember that you want this. Deeply. Stop a moment and think it through. Do you really want a belly full of food that you aren't hungry for?

Use the 1 to 10 Importance Scale This is the strong clarifying tool we saw in Chapter 4. Ask yourself, after a few deep breaths: On a scale from 1 to 10 how important is it to me to eat this food I'm not hungry for right now? On a scale from 1 to 10 how important is it to me to release weight and live out my wellness vision? Seeing that you want your healthy weight more will help you turn your attention away from the food and onto something else.[10]

Look ahead. Ask yourself, "What's going to make me feel great, now and later?" Think through the *now* and *later* parts honestly. Only you will know. If you aren't hungry, not putting anything into your stomach is going to feel great. Whatever food you're faced with will probably show up again in your lifetime. Relax and let it go.

It really is easier than you think once you don't reach for the food automatically. Permission makes it easier and easier to let things go. Feel the triumph! You can do this.

Check-in for hunger. If you are hungry, enjoy. Eat mindfully.

What About "Special" Food?

Keep reminding yourself that special foods are *not* illegal anymore. All foods are neutral. If you're not hungry, remember you can have any food you want when your body needs fuel again, and it will need fuel again. Can you save some for later? If the food can't be saved and it's a rare opportunity you may never have again, taste it with wonder! You don't have to make it a meal; a few wonderful bites will be a gift.

I recently had the chance to try several very interesting Japanese foods brought home by a friend. I wasn't hungry, but I had a lovely bite of each one and am so glad I did. That choice is what made me feel best in that unusual situation.

No matter where we are when external cues show up, we can know that we are safe between our hunger and satisfaction cues. As long as these two signals are our boundaries, we can't go wrong. And if we happen to over-eat—there is mercy. We learn from the experience and walk on down our path toward liberty.

Emotional Cues

Emotional cues aren't from the outside world but are from the very real world in our head and heart. As with external cues, emotional cues are *disconnected* from the physical needs of our body. Trying to satisfy emotional hunger with food-fuel will work *against* us and our health.

Every week in workshop I hear stories of emotional eating. We are emotional creatures and this is one of our biggest challenges. The good news is that we can learn new, effective ways of coping that will lead us to feel much better than overeating ever did and will not harm our body and mind.

Recently a very distraught friend was sharing in workshop how she had toiled for months on a major project at work. She had done the hard work, worked overtime, given 100 percent, seen it through, and in the end her new boss took the credit. That hard week of going unrecognized coincided with some other personal emotional disappointments and loneliness. Her solace was Double Stuf Oreos. As she poured her heart out, we all empathized and reassured her that she is not alone in this reaction to a very disappointing situation and that it could have been much worse. She could have committed murder. Just sharing the story was cathartic. We have all eaten to numb, to comfort, to escape, to forget.

She came in feeling like a failure and left understanding that an overeating event is a necessary part of this journey toward liberated eating. These experiences are exactly how we learn to take good care of ourselves under pressure. Through this experience she learned a lot about herself, her needs, and how she might have helped herself in other ways. She will be ready next time a crazy week happens. We all learned a lot along with her.

Remember that "Relapse" is the best school! Please hear this loud and clear. Anyone on this journey to becoming a liberated eater is going to fall back into old coping patterns sometimes. Maybe a lot at first. Change is not a straight line. We just pick ourselves up, dust ourselves off, see what we can learn, keep going and grow a little wiser for the experience.

The stumble actually makes perfect sense. When we are emotionally uncomfortable, it stands to reason that we will be looking for relief. Very often we really *do* need a way of escape. Our job now is to find a better escape route—one that will not harm us in the process of relieving us—and we can. We can find a workable solution to our discomfort that leaves us much happier than falling into a food coma. Every situation is workable.

What Am I Really Hungry For?

First let's take a look at what we really need. We know this, but after repeatedly defaulting to food for comfort, it's good to *re*-remember. Think of all the emotions we can experience in any given day. What do these emotions tell us we're hungry for?

When we're bored, we're hungry for stimulation or purpose. When we feel lonely, we're hungry for companionship. What are we hungry for when we feel weary? How often we reach for a Coke or a big shot of coffee when what we really hunger for is a nap or a few moments of quiet. When angry, we hunger for expression, understanding, and perhaps justice. When stressed, we hunger for peace. We hunger for clarity, perspective, and wisdom when we're feeling confused. When we're happy, we hunger for celebration! A leaping child-like dance or a few loud whoops would satisfy more than a pint of Ben & Jerry's and leave us feeling refreshed rather than regretful.

Food is the absolute *best* answer for physical hunger, but it's a dangerous answer for emotional hunger. You can binge all day and it will never satisfy because you can never get enough of what you're not hungry for.

Does eating *remedy* or *satisfy* any of these emotions? Did the Oreos satisfy my friend's deep disappointment? No, it added more.

But can eating *mask* these emotions? Absolutely. She felt transported while eating the Oreos. It felt as though the hurt was being crunched away with each chocolaty sweet cookie. But when the overeating was done—the feelings that started the whole eating event were still there. Loud and clear. With heavy food regret on top.

Why is turning to food so common? I mean, besides the fact that it tastes good, it's legal, and it's relatively cheap. In his book *Shrink Yourself*, Dr. Roger Gould paints this picture: ". . . the food trance . . . feels like a safe place, a bubble, a zone where you feel nurtured, loved, free from responsibility. The food trance is a place to find rest from bad feelings—it's the place where the bad feelings are actually transformed momentarily into the pleasure of eating. The food trance is an escape."

When we're eating compulsively, it feels as though time stands still. We are transported. Eating this way is such a thorough, immediate, and tactile distraction that everything else is canceled out for the moment. Eating this way can feel frenzied, desperate, and out of control—or quite peaceful. It often takes place in secret, which only adds to our feelings of isolation and brokenness. But let me assure you, you are not alone in this behavior—and you are not broken.

How can we change this pattern and find an effective and sustainable way to deal with emotional hunger? Let's look at what other choices we do have.

Chapter 16

THE FORK IN THE ROAD

Learning to Sit a While

*W*hen you're plagued by a strong, crazy, persistent urge to eat that's driven by emotions—it's right then that you are at the proverbial "fork in the road" and have at least three choices. The trick is to sit and think a moment before taking off running down the much traveled road of compulsive eating.

First, it's good to know where each of our choices will take us. One road leads to eating emotionally . . . the crazy cycle of "I feel uncomfortable, I eat, I regret." This road is well worn and easy to take but will lead us where we don't want to go.

The second choice is to get busy doing something besides eating. We can simply distract ourselves until the craving is gone. No craving lasts forever. In fact they are usually gone in about fifteen or twenty minutes. Brush your teeth, take a stroll, write a note, listen to music, sweep the patio, brush the dog, anything that is pleasant and *not* near food.

The third choice we have is to deal with the actual emotion or situation that is causing us to want to eat in the first place—to get to the bottom of it. This choice may take some courage but will relieve the source of the compulsion.

With the last two, either way, you win! You haven't taken in fuel your body doesn't need and the feeling passes. Just know that if you choose distraction the feelings may come back—depending on the situation.

Now that we know where each road will lead let's look at the crucial choice to "sit with it." When you find yourself at the Fork in the Road sitting still for about fifteen to twenty minutes is critical. Then you can identify what's driving this demanding urge to eat.

It's empowering to know that there is a moment of choice—and it is ours. Sitting at the fork gives us time to think. We are not helpless victims of a process beyond our control. We can accomplish what we want to accomplish in spite of strong urges to eat. Just the fact that you are thinking about it is big. Even if you choose to go ahead and eat this time you have already changed the usual path of immediately defaulting to food, and that is significant.

This decision to sit at the fork is the difference between *reacting* and *responding*—between things changing or remaining the same. And, these minutes of sitting with it are probably going to feel like pulling your teeth out with pliers at first. If you're like I was for thirty years, you're used to taking off down the compulsive eating road at a nice fast clip for big quick relief. Sitting still will not be something you relish. That's okay. If waiting feels terribly difficult, tell yourself that you certainly *may* decide to eat at the end of the sitting time, *but* you want to make that choice in your right mind. This puts YOU in charge instead of the compulsion.

> It's empowering to know that there is a moment of choice— and it is ours.

Being Undisturbed Has Its Challenges

I know we don't always have twenty minutes of uninterrupted time to sit. If you only have five minutes, take them. I have heard some very creative solutions: People at work getting under their desks so no one will find them for a few precious minutes, finding a quiet bathroom stall and pulling their feet up so no one knows they're there, moms sitting in the bathroom because that's the only place they can go where their kids understand they aren't to be disturbed.

When our children were young I occasionally got in our big lab's dog house for just a few minutes of solitude. It was fine even if she was home— Springer was very comforting and she never talked much. When our son found me it was the end of my solitude. It delighted him to no end to find his mother in the dog house. It became *his* hide-out of course and actually touched off a season of him eating the "cheese" out of the Kibbles & Bits. I believe this qualifies as disordered eating.

Learning How to Sit Without Judgment

Once you've found your solitude—just sit a bit. You are sitting at the Fork in the Road instead of bolting. Breathe easily and deeply. Relax. Close your eyes. Quiet your busy mind. Let yourself just BE. After a few minutes, begin to let feelings rise to the surface. See what reveals itself to you—what is behind this strong desire to eat? Do you feel stressed? Hurried? Sad? Worried? Bored? Our goal is to be still long enough to identify the feeling or the situation that is pushing our buttons. It is very important that you DO NOT JUDGE the emotions you feel—just identify them. (If nothing ever arises, don't sweat it. You have had some nice alone time and have probably been able to get back in your right mind rather than your compulsive one.)

Sometimes we've defaulted to eating so long and so quickly that we've lost touch with our real feelings. Be patient. They will probably become clear in time.

Remember, do not judge your feelings. This can seem foreign if you're prone to self-criticism as many of us are. But your feelings are just that—feelings. Feelings are not wrong in and of themselves—even strong or negative ones. In fact, they're there for a reason. They are red flags letting you know that something needs your attention. Certainly, *acting on* some of our feelings would be wrong, but the feelings themselves are not. Feelings are human. Acknowledging your feelings and being honest about them is the first step to handling them well.

If being non-judgmental is very difficult for you, try thinking of your feelings like you would think of clouds in the sky. You notice clouds for what they are but you don't judge them or try to change them. They are what they are.

Catherine, is a nurse by day and her elderly father's care-giver by night. He is grumpy to say the least, and was not a kind father during her child-hood. She rarely gets a full night's sleep since he needs assistance every two or three hours. Eating can feel like welcomed relief. When Catherine sits at the Fork in the Road, she will probably feel anger, fatigue, frustration, unappreciated—to name a few. If she judges her feelings she could falsely determine she is unloving, too easily aggravated or impatient . . . which would lead to feelings of guilt which would drain her and render her much less effective in her role as care-giver. The truth is she's an excellent and faithful care-giver, consistently choosing to be patient and kind. This is a very great love. Her feelings of frustration do not change this one bit. In fact, they make me admire her more. She can acknowledge her feelings, be honest about them, deal with them and then take good care of her father. She has done this for years. The woman is a warrior!

When we judge our feelings we cannot see them clearly. We're too busy judging to be objective or discerning. This is a self-condemning judgment that leads to shame, which often isolates, paralyzes, and blinds us from the truth. Compulsive overeating is simply not a place for shame. Your overeating makes perfect sense when you stop judging it and begin to understand it. Showing yourself mercy rather than delivering judgment is as essential to this process of change as breath is to life.

By the way, if you realize that what you are feeling is anger, it is helpful to know that *anger is often a secondary emotion*. There is often an emotion underneath our anger. Disappointment, fear, feeling taken for granted, betrayal, hurt, etc. It may be beneficial to sit a bit longer and see if there is something below the feeling of anger.

One other thing to keep in mind: When we *deny* our feelings the feelings and their effects do not go away. They are simply not acknowledged. The feelings will continue to push from behind to search for the relief your mind and body need. Highly respected therapist Kay Arnold explains it this way: "Just as there isn't closeness in a marriage without vulnerability and sensitivity to the emotions of each partner, there may also be no closeness to self without awareness of our own emotions, sensitivities and vulnerabilities. Since some of us learned early in life to bottle up and shut down the expression of emotion, there may be genuine fear that the expression or mention of those emotions might result in a never-ending, out of control cascade of uncomfortable sensations. It is only after experiencing those very intense emotions *with safe people* that we become comfortable with our authentic selves, emotions and all."

After sitting at the Fork in the Road for a while you will be able to decide what's next. Do you want to distract yourself and then see what happens? Do you want to deal with the real issue? Do you want to go ahead and eat? This is completely up to YOU. Each of these choices has pros and cons. It is very interesting to note what happens when you've had time to sit and think and experience feelings—you go from the crazy intensity of the urge to devour food to thinking clearly. When that happens, you can make the best choice for yourself.

The Fork in the Road came alive for me in an experience I had not long after we had became empty nesters. For about two weeks I had fought with a raging desire to eat everything sweet and greasy I could find. It had been a busy two weeks—lots of distractions. Still, I wanted cookies and pizza and donuts and candy corn (I don't even like candy corn). I wanted it all, fast and in large quantities. I had been reasonably recovered from crazy eating for five or six years by this time so it seemed weird to feel so strongly compulsive again for weeks. One afternoon I was so emotionally exhausted that I decided to just sit still a while and see what in the world was going on. I sat on the floor in my closet just because it seemed kind of dark and reverent—plus I couldn't see all the stuff I needed to do if I was in there. I sat a few minutes feeling nothing in particular. As I sat still and quiet I slowly began to feel sad. The longer I sat the sadder I felt. I wasn't sure why so I sat some more. It wasn't long before it became abundantly clear that I missed my kids. The silence in the house was very loud all of a sudden. I wouldn't wish them back home for anything. We loved watching them become adults—but I still missed them. Their presence. The hair balls on the bathroom floor. Smelly, grassy cleats and goalie gloves. Rollers and girl stuff on the bathroom counters. Kate's books and Em's drawing pencils and J's soccer balls. And the noise—loud laughter and slamming drawers and feet up and down the stairs. I just plain missed them. Wasn't long before the tears came. Those good kinds of tears that come from somewhere deep and flow clean and unhindered. I laid on each of their beds and smelled their pillows and cried some more. The tears eventually went from sad tears to thankful tears and then ran their course and went away. And, I kid you not (pardon the pun), the nagging desire to constantly eat cookies went with them. I wasn't hungry for vanilla sandwich cookies after all. I was hungry for a good cry. And it was very, very satisfying.

So, in this case it was dealt with. At other times distracting yourself will be the best thing. Some uncomfortable feelings are short lived—there isn't something long term to deal with. Every now and then it may even be a fine choice to go ahead and eat. Remember my warrior friend, Catherine. One especially long and difficult night her father was particularly belligerent and impossible. After many hours of difficult behavior and messes and work that most of us never endure, she decided that having survived the night without losing her sanity, hungry or not, she was treating herself to a fast food breakfast. The coming reward helped her survive, and indeed they both made it through the long night. She left as the sun came up, made her way to the drive-thru and sat in her car—alone—in the blessed quiet—and slowly savored her breakfast. Bravo!

Now, here is a very important thing to remember. The moment of choice will come many times over the course of your journey toward liberated eating. And no one I know chooses *not* to eat every single time. Change is not about perfection. It's about persistence. When you choose not to eat— remember how it feels. This gives you strength for the next battle. *But*, when you go ahead and eat, even if you eat compulsively—know this: the thinking process you have just gone through, the wrestling with your choices, is very significant. It is forward motion. It is changing things. Just *thinking* about it rather than immediately falling headlong into the food at 120 miles per hour is change! Big change. This is new and it is good and it is significant. You are changing deep pathways.

Well, as you can see, this tool we call The Fork in the Road is not for the faint of heart. We must summon our courage here. You can also see how powerful it is. We can break our long-standing patterns. We can change our course. We can have the health and peace we have wanted for so long. We can accomplish what we want to accomplish, in spite of our feelings.

When we stop covering up our emotions with food, we eventually begin to see clearly and find the real answers to the real questions.

Everybody Needs a Team

When Kay mentioned the importance of experiencing our intense emotions with safe people she touched on an essential component of support.

We know that almost no one makes a significant life-change alone. Change takes Truth, Time, Tools and Team: a trustworthy solution, time to practice our new ways, effective tools for different situations and a team that supports us and fits our unique needs.

As I look back over my years of teaching and coaching, I see that this can look many different ways for different people. It's exciting to think about building a team that will support you on your journey.

Rick has recently dropped below 400 pounds for the first time in twenty years. He has released 160 pounds so far. What a joy to celebrate with him! He has gone through workshop twice and is well on his mindful eating journey. He regularly attends a Recovery Group at his church, has good friends to call on and a wise counselor. He says, "Workshop gave me the path and tools I need, my counselor opened my eyes and through Celebrate Recovery, Jesus gave me the strength to change." This is a great description of the right team for him.

Pat has fiercely struggled for years with discouraging physical pain, depression, fatigue and compulsive bingeing. She has made great strides as she has embraced the idea of developing the right team for herself. She put it this way, "Something good is happening! Between liberated eating workshop, counseling, B12 shots, vitamins, backing off my diet drinks, and water aerobics 3-4 times a week, I am pain-free most days with no sugar cravings. Haven't binged in months. It's SO nice not to feel like food is controlling my life. I'm finally running the show again."

Each of us can get the support we need to move forward. Some need a small support team and some a large one. Some possibilities are an accountability/ encouragement buddy or group, liberated eating workshop, organizations such as Celebrate Recovery or YMCA groups, a nurse practitioner, doctor or other health professional, fitness trainer, dietician, nutritionist, diabetes support group, a walking buddy, prayer partner and others. Just make sure that the people you choose are on the same page about a non-diet approach to eating as you are. You may have to introduce some people to the principles of Liberated Eating. Most people are open to new ideas and will appreciate the insight. Make sure you gather a team that is encouraging, positive and believes that you can accomplish what you want to accomplish in spite of your obstacles.

You will know what kind of support you need as you think, learn, and become more and more intuitive and honest with yourself. You may talk it through with a coach or friend but ultimately you will know what you need—and in time you will be on someone else's team. Now that's exciting!

Chapter 17

COPING WITH EMOTIONS

Choosing Not to Stuff it Down With Food

*J*t is not uncommon for people who struggle with food to be nurturers—people who serve, who give others a lot of grace but do not extend it to themselves. A highly respected eating disorder specialist once told me that the people she works with are often "the best and the brightest," high achievers holding themselves to very high standards with little or no room for mistakes.

It is also not uncommon for people who struggle with their relationship with food to be on the passive end of the passive-assertive spectrum. They have much they wish to say but instead of saying it, remain silent and often turn to food as a substitute for expression. In a sense they are using food to stuff down their words. Recently I was discussing this with a therapist who said that often passive people have or have had someone significant in their life who is aggressive or overbearing. Because of this they confuse the good qualities of being assertive with the negative qualities of being aggressive. They don't want to be aggressive, since this doesn't hold good memories for them. They don't wish to resemble the bully in their life. The danger here is letting the pendulum swing too far in the other direction, becoming passive and frustrated and then turning to food for relief.

I like this definition by psychologists Robert Alberti and Michael Emmons: Assertive behavior is "behavior which enables a person to act in his own best interests, to stand up for himself without undue anxiety, to express his honest feelings comfortably, or to exercise his own rights without denying the rights of others."

Assertive and *aggressive* are not the same thing. The good news is that we can certainly learn how to become more assertive if we wish to. Getting help in this area is a great gift to give yourself and those who love you.[11]

Be Prepared for "Right" to Feel "Wrong" at First

Over the years, many of us have become very comfortable with our excessive, tranquilizing emotional eating. There is a deep and well-worn path to reach for food automatically. It feels good and safe and familiar.

Eating emotionally will feel very "right" and choosing *not* to do it may feel very "wrong" at first.

Your feelings will not understand why you are not tranquilizing them as usual. Get ready for them to demand what they're used to. We must be willing to tolerate the intense drive to overeat. And we can. It will not last forever. Every time we wait for true hunger instead of feeding our emotions, we get closer and closer to normalizing our relationship with food.

Another thing to recognize is that when you're no longer eating emotionally, you will probably begin to feel the feelings you used to cover up with food. You may find that you're experiencing more feelings than you are used to—comfortable and uncomfortable ones. Some things may become clear that were not clear before. When we are no longer distracting ourselves with food, we free up emotional space for what is authentic.

I've seen people realize they hate their job and need to find a new one; admit to themselves and others that they are being mistreated; find new interests, ministries, and passions; and mend fences with friends and family. Some people cry a lot for a time and

> Your feelings will not understand why you are not tranquilizing them as usual. Get ready for them to demand what they're used to.

soon feel a huge weight off their shoulders that had been there so long they thought it was normal. My friend Teresa said, "Now that I'm not regularly stuffing my emotions with food, I cry more and laugh more than I ever have, and I love it—I feel more alive!" Others have said that their family and friends want to know what has happened to them—they just seem more alive. I have watched in wonder as people literally transform week after week as they become more and more free. Often their face begins to relax and glow with life. We're not only numbing our feelings when we eat emotionally; we are often numbing our true selves. Change is exciting and so worth the courageous work it takes!

This Core Belief reminds us that we can indeed effectively cope with our physical and emotional hunger in ways that bring vibrant strength to our health and our heart.

 Core Belief

HANDLE EMOTIONS WITHOUT USING FOOD

I can deal with my emotions without using food. Food is the best solution for hunger. It is not an effective solution for stress, boredom, happiness, anger, etc. I am very capable of finding appropriate solutions.

So what do we do with all these emotions if we aren't stuffing them anymore? As I have the privilege of walking alongside people on this journey I learn a lot from them. Here are some of the things people do to cope with their emotions rather than turn to food. You will find what works best for you.

Coping well with **STRESS:** Take a walk, run, breathe deeply, have a relaxing bath, meditate, pray, get a massage, play something vigorous, visit the firing range, dance, stretch or do yoga, remember "this too shall pass," rearrange furniture, mow, clean things, exercise, work a puzzle, make a list.

Coping well with **ANGER:** Hit something you can't hurt, start kick-boxing, walk fast, walk slow, exercise vigorously, take up clogging, watch a funny movie, journal, go ahead and cry or scream, talk it out with a trusted counselor or friend—or your dog—as you look for a possible resolution.

Coping well with **BOREDOM:** Leave the house, walk around the block and find a neighbor to visit, learn a second language, start that book you've always wanted to write, go play (just jump in and you'll remember how), go help someone do something, swing at your nearest park, call an elderly friend, revisit that long-lost hobby or start a new one, put on loud music and tackle a project or chore, dance, make something fun and give it away, find your crayons and color with a child, do one thing that you would be glad you did.

Coping well with HAPPINESS: Share it if you can, run, walk, dance, sing a song real loud, take a drive with the windows down and the music up, finger paint, skip, hula hoop, wear a silly hat, do a Tarzan yell, roll down a grassy hill, jump on a trampoline.

Coping well with FATIGUE: Sit quietly and breathe deeply, close your eyes for five or ten minutes (in a dark room if you can), put your feet up and read a magazine, take a nap, read an enjoyable book that isn't for your self-improvement, stretch, take a walk while you breathe relaxingly.

Coping well with CONFUSION: Get outside your own head and talk to a wise and safe person, breathe, pray, walk briskly, ask questions, write about or draw a diagram of your thoughts.

Coping well with LONELINESS: Do some research on what safe and positive groups of people gather in your area and then join a fellowship of people who share similar interests with you, reconnect with old friends or family, get a pet, start a book club.

Coping well with SADNESS: Go ahead and cry, walk, express the sadness to someone you trust, express it through painting or writing, hike in a place very pleasant to you, wrap up in a soft blanket and have a cup of tea, comfort someone else, swing, get a massage.

Many of these things overlap and will work well for other emotions. *The important thing is to fill the place that food used to take with something helpful.* If we take the food out and don't put something else in that place it will be difficult not to fall back into old familiar patterns.

Keep in mind that it's possible that food has masked some very significant issues in our lives. I'm a huge fan of finding wise, professional counsel for issues that can threaten my long-term health and wellness or that of my family. Please don't hesitate to find the help you might need so you can flourish.

Once you begin to answer your emotions with effective solutions and expressions, you will begin to feel more peaceful, more in charge and less anxious. You are very capable of taking good care of yourself and finding the help and answers you're looking for—the ones that will take you where you want to go with your health.

Chapter 18

WHO'S DRIVING THIS BUS ANYWAY?

You Get to Choose

After years of emotional eating and roller-coaster dieting, doesn't it make sense that we might feel shaky about our ability to live peacefully with food and our bodies? As we make our way along this new journey toward health, we may encounter some fear—fear that this mindful/intuitive eating thing won't work either.

This fear feels especially founded when we hear negative, discouraging and crazy thoughts swirling around in our head. Each one of us can want and think many conflicting things at the same time. The thing to remember is that this is perfectly normal. Just because the thoughts are there doesn't mean that they're in charge. The good news is we don't have to have every thought under control and perfectly congruent before we can move forward and reach our goals.

A helpful exercise is to imagine a bus trip. This trip represents your journey with food. It points out your ability to allow negative thoughts to be present in your head without having to act on them, while still moving forward.

There are many different passengers on the bus; they represent the thoughts we each have flying through our heads at any given time. But where the bus ends up depends on who's driving. The people on the bus (the thoughts in our head) may all want to go different places—but the driver is going to take the bus where he or she wants to go.

There is only one driver. The driver is YOU, in your right mind, headed in the direction you truly wish to go . . . toward your wellness vision. Let's take a ride on my bus to see what this might look like.

Hop aboard! You will notice Liberated Me in the driver's seat—but I am certainly not alone.

- Sitting a few rows behind the driver and being very vocal is Food-Focused Cindy. She wants to bake a batch of oatmeal cookies with pecans and chocolate chips and eat half the dough while they bake and then devour a pile of hot cookies with reckless abandon as soon as they come out of the oven, probably burning her tongue. This Me wants to turn the bus toward the grocery store so she can run in and get some chocolate chips.
- Unrealistic Cindy wants to be very, very thin after seeing a fit looking fifty-something woman in a movie. This Me wants to drive the bus toward an extreme solution, like fasting for five days or swearing off sugar for the rest of the month. Both these Me's are yelling their requests at the driver.
- Then there's Melancholy Me from college. She's gained forty-plus pounds in just a few months and is miserable and out of control. She's sitting in the back of the bus, alone, slowly eating Cowboy Cookies from Safeway as she painfully contemplates starting a new diet on Monday. She doesn't really care where this bus is going as long as she can hide and eat her cookies.
- Trying to isolate herself in the middle of the bus is Restrictive Me. She's adding up calories in her head because she thinks she might've overdone it at lunch. This thought makes her agitated and fearful of gaining a pound. Restrictive Me wants to drive the bus to the bookstore so she can get that new book on counting calories, carbs, points, and fat grams. Having all this info at her fingertips just might make her behave.
- Close by is Compulsive Me—she's lost in a recurring thought loop that vacillates between horribly regretting that bag of Fritos she ate late last night and desperately wanting to finish off the second bag in the pantry as soon as she gets home. I mean, if they're all gone she can forget about them, right?

- A few rows back is Critical Me, feeling very smug and justified. She's scrutinizing her body and berating herself for not being thinner. The inner dialogue goes something like this: "You're a blimp," "Your thighs look like hams," "You're disgusting." She has a long list of practiced insults. Somewhere in the back of her mind she thinks these criticisms might just motivate her to change—even though this strategy has never worked before. She wants to drive the bus straight to (and away from) the closest mirror.
- Whiney Me is sitting right behind the driver complaining out loud about even having to think about this at all. A lot of lucky people never give this food-fat thing a thought. It's just not fair! She looks tired and unpleasant. No one wants to sit next to her.
- In the back of the bus not far from Melancholy, being pitifully obnoxious, is Hopeless Me, convincing herself nothing will ever work. She feels perfectly powerless to change anything—which, to be honest, is actually rather comforting because then she's off the hook. Might as well not even try.

Now all of these passengers and more are on my bus, and *all* of them want to drive. *All* of them think they know exactly where we need to go.

Here's the good news: I get to decide who's going to drive my bus! The other passengers may come and go. And they don't have to be kicked off in order for me to reach my destination.

I can make a conscious decision that the Me who is driving the bus is the Me who's headed for my best health and energy. This Me has her eyes on the road, every now and then checking the map to make sure we're on course. She makes sure she has some support for the journey and checks in with others who have traveled this road before. This Me is looking toward the future. She's got her eye on her destination and is mindful of the next few miles as well. Yes, she can hear the chatter in the back, occasionally looking in the rearview mirror and acknowledging what's going on. At times she may be tempted to join in the conversation, but she knows it would be fruitless.

> We don't have to have every thought under control and perfectly congruent before we can move forward and reach our goals.

The driver doesn't have to judge or change the other people on the bus. This would just use up precious energy and accomplish nothing. She accepts each of them for who they are but is not affected by their opinions. The driver also doesn't think that she has to argue with them or stop the bus and wrestle each one off before she can move on. She lets them be and moves ahead.

The driver knows where she's going, has done her homework about the best route, and is allowing for some flexibility along the way. She knows it will take some time, but she will reach her destination.

And here's the really cool thing: as the bus gets closer and closer to the goal, the other passengers begin to see the light, the reason for going this way, the good sense in it—and one by one they begin to get on board with the driver. By the time they arrive they might even be singing a few cheesy rounds of "The Wheels on the Bus Go 'Round and 'Round."

Choosing How You Think

It Really Matters

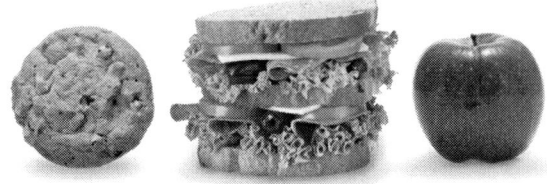

KNOW THY BRAIN

Both of Them

When you feel that overwhelming, crazy-intense urge to compulsively overeat, knowing how your brain works will help you get back in charge. Your brain is an amazingly complex universe. For our purposes we will *greatly* simplify it into two parts.

Our high executive functioning brain is a grown-up. It thinks ahead, considers consequences, critiques, evaluates, etc. Living with this practical grown-up brain is a childish brain. If you're like me you are very familiar with the impulsive youngster living in your brain. It wants what it wants when it wants it! No thought of responsibility, consequences, or tomorrow.

The child in our brain believes, and for good reason, that if it screams long enough and loud enough the grown-up will eventfully wear down, wear out and give in—anything to stop that blasted noise! The more we've given in lately the more power the child thinks it has. And here's the hard part: Guess who is the loudest when you're in pain, scared, stressed or uncomfortable. Yep, the small child in your brain.

When you're at your worst . . . the child is at its best. It starts by screaming for a two-pound bag of M&Ms. If that doesn't work, it screams louder and adds a Wendy's Frosty to the list—whichever is quickest. And while we're at the drive-thru, how about a double bacon cheeseburger and large fries? *We're in pain here! We'll worry about details later! This is serious—give me my Frosty!!!*

Now, here's the kicker, once you've given in and eaten the large bag of M&Ms and the super-sized meal—lo and behold, your grown-up brain pipes up and criticizes you *after the fact.* "How could you have done this again? You're so weak. What is wrong with you? You're hopeless!"

Really? Where was my grown-up brain when all that yelling was going on? It was temporarily shut out of the discussion. When we're stressed or scared, there is a trap door between our grown-up brain and our child brain[12] that slams shut temporarily—so the child is driving the bus . . . and we all know how well that works.

Now, here's the really good news. With enough support, insight, and practice the grown-up brain can be in charge. Absolutely. Just like in real life, adults can lead no matter how loud the child screams. The trick is to recognize when it's the child who is screaming and then choose not to let it lead. Ear plugs and a calm smile go a long way in tolerating the demanding tantrum. Your grown-up brain can overrule the upset child. That's exciting!

> With enough support, insight, and practice the grown-up brain can be in charge. Absolutely.

The Fork in the Road is a powerful tool for giving your grown-up brain the last word. Here's the cool thing. The desire to eat emotionally will dim as you learn other ways of coping. This is challenging in the beginning because you are changing things, but it will get easier and easier with practice. We can stop the crazy-eating cycle.

As we pause and sit a while before running to food, as we begin to summon the courage to stop defaulting to food—new and wonderful things begin to grow. When we begin to do some things differently we begin to see that *life really can be different!* Change begets change.

Chapter 20

WAYS OF THINKING
TO ESCORT OUT

Self-Criticism, Negation
and All-or-Nothing Thinking

There are certain ways of thinking that, if allowed to lead, will take us farther and farther from our best health. Let's identify three of these and begin to root them out permanently.

Firing the Critical Judge

Those of us who have struggled with food often struggle with self-criticism as well. And it makes sense. Overeating leads to self-criticism because we feel powerless against the compulsive force. Dieting leads us to criticize ourselves because we think we're too weak to "stick to it."

If we don't understand what's going on we'll think we deserve this criticism and dutifully dish it out in big, toxic servings inside our own heads—which only leads to feeling more helpless and defeated. This isn't true, but when we believe it's true, we will act as if it is. For many of us this creates a gut-wrenching, hope-killing downward spiral.

Of course we now know that diets are not sustainable (it's the diet that's flawed, not you) and that compulsive overeating is a normal response to diet-deprivation. However, even with this knowledge it's easy to continue to live in self-criticism. This, like overeating, can feel normal after years of practice.

Now your important task is to silence the critical judge in your head and become the curious observer instead. This allows you to evaluate your eating behavior from a neutral place—like a non-biased scientist. Then you can learn from your mistakes. Adopting this core belief is powerful!

 Core Belief

FIRE THE CRITICAL JUDGE

I am a curious observer—not a critical judge—of my eating behavior. I do not allow negative, self-condemning thoughts which keep me from moving forward. I have learned to be merciful with myself, even when I don't make the best choices. I learn from these missteps.

Please understand why this is so important: The latest brain research shows us what we already know from life experience. Our high-executive functioning brain uses a huge amount of energy when we're self-criticizing. We become sidetracked from positive, proactive, and effective thinking and use up all our energy being angry and negative. It's a monumental waste of good brain power!

Self-acceptance and *self-respect*, however, lead to creative solution finding and the courage to change. With acceptance and respect come hope and strength.

Imagine that you're out in the backyard with a child who is criticizing herself for struggling with riding a bicycle, which is proving to be quite a challenge for her. You know that she's done hard things before; she's very capable and can certainly accomplish this goal and more . . . but *she* doesn't believe it. On this subject she has convinced herself that she's incapable.

What would a caring adult say to this child? Most would empathize with the challenge and encourage her. "It will be worth all this hard work. Remember the time you . . . ? You kept on and you got it! You will get this too."

What do you predict will happen if she keeps berating herself?

What if she accepts her need to continue to practice?

What if she has mercy on herself when she falls, gets back on, keeps trying, and begins to trust that she can indeed learn to ride her bike? What if she even begins to have a sense of humor about the process? What if she accepts the support offered and keeps working on it? You and I both know that this young lady will eventually be flying up and down the street and having the time of her life!

You are this child. You are more than capable of living well with food. You are more than capable of taking good care of yourself and your body—of reaching and sustaining the comfortable weight and energy you desire. Give yourself the same grace and encouragement that you would offer to this girl moping beside her bicycle.

In the same way, when you hear critical thoughts in your head, stop yourself on the spot. Keep in mind that the criticism will be in your own voice—it will sound perfectly normal so have your ear tuned to *the message.* When you recognize the negative self-talk, stop it, acknowledge that it is not the truth, and remind yourself that you will not tolerate these thoughts about yourself. This isn't just pie-in-the-sky positive thinking. It's a vitally important next step; it's rooting out old destructive lies with truth.

It has been estimated that over 90 percent of the thoughts we think are the same ones we thought yesterday. This alone is a great reason to begin to say kind things to yourself.

Now comes a very important step. You must replace the "old recordings" with some new ones. If you don't, those old critical thoughts will move right back in and make themselves at home where they've been comfortable for quite some time.

You will need to find what truths and phrases resonate with you. It may be an encouraging phrase, song or thought from someone you have known. It may be a quote, poem or verse that sums up the truth you wish to take root in your core.

Many years ago I went on a retreat where the speaker's theme was "You are a person of worth, worthy of respect and love. Even from yourself." This was a new concept to me at the time. It shook me and shaped me. This is one I still go to. I also repeat our self-efficacy statement often: "I can accomplish what I want to accomplish in spite of obstacles."

It's vital that you have this thought ready so when you catch yourself in the act of self-criticizing you can stop it and choose life-giving thoughts instead.

Powerful, Practical Self-Criticism Busters

While we are working on the stuff that goes on in our heads, let's take a look at a few practical things we can do that will help us quiet self-criticism from the outside.

First, consider getting rid of your scales. Yes . . . you read this correctly. Consider not weighing regularly. If that thought makes you hyperventilate then how about putting it in the attic for a few weeks. It's just a machine. It doesn't know you or how much salt you ate last night. Your weight can fluctuate greatly from day to day or as you move the scale around on the bathroom floor. Come on . . . we've all done it. At least begin to pay very close attention to what stepping on the scales does to you. What is the dialogue that goes on in your mind after you step off? If it leads you to be critical (or permissive), please consider doing this part of your life differently.

And think about this: that machine does not help you connect with your body—which is one of your goals. Your body, energy, and clothes will intuitively tell you everything you need to know. I know very few people for whom the scales are a helpful tool. Please be very honest with yourself about what conversation takes place in your head after stepping on them.

Second, have some FUN! It is much easier to think proactively when you're regularly producing endorphins in your brain and enjoying yourself. No wonder so many of us struggle with food—we're waiting to live until after we "lose this weight." Start living the way you want to live now and you will be *life*-focused rather than *food*-focused. You are fully *you* right now. Please don't miss a moment of being you waiting to be you when you "get thinner." Choose to enjoy your life now.

Let this sink in . . .
You do not become more valuable when you lose weight.
You just feel better.

Third, spend more time hanging out with positive, respectful people. I know this may take some courage. Sometimes there are people in our lives who can be negative, skeptical, and discouraging. These people can range from mildly irritating to danger- ously toxic. We must decide what we are going to do about this. We are in charge of the influences we allow into our lives. We are in charge of setting boundaries that keep the good stuff in and the bad stuff out. There is plenty of good help available when it comes to learning how to set healthy bound- aries. Please do not hesitate to get help if you need it.

> Start living the way you want to live now and you will be *life*-focused rather than *food*-focused. You are fully *you* right now.

You can decide not to be derailed by anyone's words. Their opinion does not change your plans or dreams. Don't let anything or anyone sidetrack you from your health goals.

Set your face like a flint on your destination—your health destiny. It is yours for the taking.

Stop Telling Yourself to Stop (Negation)

I know this sounds crazy, but research teaches us that your deepest brain cannot hear "not." If you walk into a Mexican restaurant, saying to yourself as you walk in, "I am *not* going to stuff myself tonight. I am *not*! I am *not* going to walk out of here feeling miserable again like last time!" your brain is hearing, "I am going to stuff myself tonight. I am! I am going to walk out of here feeling miserable again just like last time!" And guess what? You probably will.

Now before you write this off, just think about this a minute. How many times have you yelled, "Don't slam that door!" only to hear a slam. But when someone says in a quiet tone, "Close the door gently," no slam. This is pow- erful stuff right here. You can use this when you're around food. Tell yourself what you *are* going to do—instead of what you are *not* going to do. Try some of these phrases on for size next time you go to a food-filled event:

- I'm going to enjoy a slow and relaxed meal tonight. I am going to eat the best bites first and savor each one.
- I'm going as a connoisseur—looking everything over, choosing exactly what I want, and fully enjoying every bite.

- This is going to be a peaceful evening. I am going to be fully present and enjoy the conversation, the meal, and the moment.

You can do this—and it's way more fun than thinking about what you are *not* supposed to do.

All-or-Nothing Thinking

Another way of thinking that will sabotage our forward momentum is all-or-nothing thinking. This is born out of our dieting experience. When we were dieting, there were "good" foods and "bad" foods. We were good when we ate only good foods and we were bad if we took one bite of a bad food. We were living under a diet-dictator and we obeyed *all* the rules or we failed. Dieting is pass or fail, black or white, success or failure, all or nothing. It's this kind of harsh, inflexible rule following that eventually overrides our common sense so that we actually believe we should either eat none of it or . . . a ton of it!

How many times have you done this? You're on a diet, minding your own business, eating by the rules. Then along comes Valentine's Day or Easter or the Super Bowl—doesn't matter what it is, there's just a lot of "special" food attached to it. You, wretched soul that you are, crumble under the strain and dare to eat a Reese's Peanut Butter egg or tree or bunny or heart. These specially shaped Reese's are manufactured in hell just to tempt us. I know this is true because there is more of that peanut butter stuff in them and this is devilishly diabolical.

The act of eating the forbidden thing sends you into a tailspin of overeating and eventually into confused despair . . . again.

The problem here is not that you ate the Reese's. Not even close. The problem is what you *think* about eating the Reese's.

The problem is the all-or-nothing thinking that dieting produces. You can't have any because it is illegal. If you do eat even one bite then you have broken the sacred diet law. You are "bad," and if you're already bad you might as well go all out and eat *all* of it. There is no gray area, no moderation, no room for "a few." This kind of thinking overrules our usual common sense. It's none of the pie or all of the pie. It's none of the fries or a super-duper biggy size. It's perfection or a complete train wreck.

It is exactly this scenario that has caused most of our weight gain over the years. "Normal," intuitive eaters eat Reese's and pie and fries sometimes, and they eat until they are satisfied, not ill. Can you see what's going on here?

We need a drastic change—a complete paradigm shift—a new world view for our food life. We can leave the cult and step into sanity; we can go from merciless law to life-giving liberty. It's time to look at this with fresh new eyes.

Put all-or-nothing on a scale from zero to ten. "Nothing" is zero and "all" is ten. Notice that there is not just zero or ten on this scale. There is one, two, three, four, five, six, seven, eight, and nine. We have a lot of other choices besides zero or ten. What if we look at all-or-nothing as black and white? There's not just black and white; there are countless shades of grays in between.

What if over the years we had understood that we had many choices rather than all of it or none of it? What if, when we thought we'd "blown it," we had realized that we could have enjoyed four cookies or six cookies rather than none of them or the whole package?

What if, *now* that we're becoming liberated eaters, we think it through and know that, even if we choose to eat when we're not hungry, it doesn't mean we have to eat till we're sick? There is no law to break.

Begin to trust yourself with the gray area, with moderation, with one through nine, with a little too much instead of a lot too much. Begin to believe that you can indeed self-govern and that it doesn't have to be done perfectly. Begin to understand that when you don't do it perfectly it doesn't have to end in a train wreck.

You can be trusted to be reasonable.

Chapter 21

WAYS OF THINKING
TO INVITE IN

A Kind Voice, Respect Your Body Now, Think Yes

*W*e've just looked at some thought patterns that will harm our progress and we're escorting them *out*. Now let's look at a few ways of thinking that will bring the change we want and invite them *in*.

Choose a Tone That Invites Change

When you've had a bad time with food, intentionally choose a kind voice to accompany the conversation in your head. Think of a gentle, loving grandparent. Make one up if you didn't have one.

An impatient adult might snap, "You better shape up right now! You're in big trouble!" But a wise grandmother (in an ideal world) would notice that you aren't at your best. She would know that you're already disappointed with yourself and need compassion. She calls you over, pulls you close and says, "Hey, Love, you aren't quite yourself today. Is anything bothering you? Did something happen at school?" She assumes the best about you and wants to find out what is behind your behavior.

This wise grandmother isn't going to ignore harmful behavior, but she will look at the *why* before the *what*. This kind of response will often melt a child and lead to important understanding and growth. The demand to "shape up or ship out" often causes withdrawal and shame.

When you've overeaten—choose your tone carefully. Use your Grandmom voice. Choose compassion—even if it feels weird at first. Compassion, by the way, is not the same thing as just being nice. You can be nice to someone you don't care one whit about. True compassion is one of the most powerful forces on earth, or anywhere else for that matter. Compassion stops the tirade, opens the way for reflection which opens the way for understanding which opens the way for real and permanent change.

In case this feels too mushy and you're afraid you might not do any changing if you're kind to yourself—let's think this through . . .

- When you use a harsh and judgmental tone with yourself it is with the assumption that you've been bad and you deserve punishment. Punishment is not about change or improvement. It's about payback and usually leads to resignation, discouragement, anger and/or shame.
- True compassion wants your highest good therefore it would not choose to be permissive. It cares enough to discipline when it's needed. The purpose of discipline is to bring you to your very best. When you are kind to yourself you can calm down, think through what just happened and figure out how to change things.

Bottom line: Stop berating yourself. If discouragement and condemnation worked you wouldn't be reading this book.

You Gotta Value That Body Before You Can Change It

Most of us who have struggled with food have struggled with our body too. We desperately want it to be different. We've berated it and hated it, judged it and begrudged it. And all the while our bodies have stuck with us even though we've starved them, stuffed them, mocked them, medicated them, over-exercised them, or made them be sedentary against their will.

Most of us have been locked in this epic body-battle for far too long and are soul-weary with the struggle. Would you, right now, do something you may never have dreamed of doing? Consider the possibility that you have been fighting with the wrong enemy. What if your body is actually one of your biggest advocates? What if the two of you become allies rather than adversaries? What if you stop criticizing and begin to work together arm in arm? What might happen then?

It's easy to see why we have come to see our bodies as a big part of our problem. The pressure to be thin in our image-saturated culture is relentless. We see countless pictures day in and day out of "perfect," pencil-thin people. And even though we all know that the *perfection* is highly manufactured we can still feel uncomfortable with our own bodies in comparison. Seventy-eight percent of seventeen year old girls are dissatisfied with their bodies now and the number is growing. How many of us would love to have our seventeen year old body again! The average American model is 5' 11" and 117 pounds. Read that again . . . 117 pounds at almost 6 feet tall. If you saw this poor girl in Haiti you would rush to her aid! It is time to stop the insanity—at least in our own lives.

No matter what size you may be right now, please lay down your tired weapons of condemnation, relinquish the striving, take a deep breath and decide to step completely out of the battle for thinness and step into the joy of living fully, healthfully and freely out of the only body you will ever have.

Think about this: your best memories were experienced through that body you live in right now. The most fun you've ever had was possible because of your body. The last thing you saw that took your breath away was seen through those eyes in that body. The most moving music you've ever heard went through those ears of yours. The dearest expression of love you've ever given or received was given and received through that body. That body is not you, but it is the vessel that houses you and has been your constant companion. It was with you when you arrived and it will be with you when you leave. That body is something to be revered and respected.

 Core Belief

RESPECT YOUR BODY

I respect my body and am very grateful for it. It is my constant companion. I have stopped wanting it to be perfect, and I now value my body exactly as it is.

How you choose to think about your body is key to moving forward into the comfortable health and weight you so desire. Please hear this loud and clear: most of the people you think are living in perfect bodies are no more satisfied than you or I. This is a shocking truth.

Kay Arnold, a therapist with decades of experience, put it this way: "I have counseled slender, drop-dead-gorgeous beauty-teens; lovely, healthy young adults; attractive inside and out middle-aged women and men. The most common verbal thread has been 'I hate my body . . . I hate how I look.' I have concluded there is not a size that makes someone love him- or herself. It is a choice to love your body as you are, as you continue to move through life's phases." Did you hear that: *There is not a size that makes someone love him- or herself.*

Please understand, people who do not accept their body *where it is right now* (or worse, hate it) have a very hard time living in a way that will make things better.

Here's the BIG truth: If berating our bodies helped, we would all have been the weight we desire a long time ago!

I know this can feel very scary but the strange irony is that when you come to accept, honor, and respect your body just as it is—flaws and all—you then open the way for real change. When you value something, you take good care of it. When you don't value something, you probably won't.

Studies[13] find that people who are accepting and appreciative of their bodies *as they are* have much more success in reaching their health goals than those who are not.

Many people are rethinking their demand for "very-thinness." They are turning their energies to finding and keeping good health. They are getting on with their lives and enjoying it! Once they stop demanding thinness and start enjoying living in their healthy body, they experience a wonderful peace. Many release weight once they stop obsessing about "losing weight."

I'm afraid there's no way around it . . . you have to start liking yourself.

LADIES, LET US LEAVE A LASTING LEGACY

After years of walking alongside women of all ages, from teenagers to those in their eighties, it is very clear that one of the greatest gifts we can give to those younger than ourselves is the gift of valuing our body at every age and stage. For younger women to see us age gracefully, embrace and enjoy our wrinkles and changes, walk with confidence and joy, laugh easily, and stay as active and vibrant as our health will allow—to intentionally choose not to give off the distinct message that we wish we were "young again"—*this*, ladies, is one of our greatest gifts possible to those coming behind.

> What if your body is actually one of your biggest advocates? What if the two of you become allies rather than adversaries?

Love your thirties and forties. Flaunt your fifties and sixties. Enjoy your seventies and eighties with reckless abandon. Be proud of your nineties and beyond. Make us wish we were YOUR age! A dear friend of mine just passed away at 114. She embraced each year with gusto!

May we pass on the priceless legacy of *beauty and gratitude at every age*, inside and out. Those coming behind us just might escape the badgering of the relentless youth-worshiping media if they see us, in large numbers, growing more vibrant and alive with each passing year.

It's not about the number on the scale or the year on the birth certificate. It is about genuine, grateful joy.

This is noble work.

Thoughtfully Think About the Thoughts You're Thinking

Many wise counselors have shared this: Our *thoughts* lead to our *feelings*. Our *feelings* lead to our *behaviors*. Our *behaviors* lead to the *results* we want or the *consequences* we don't want.

What we *think* determines our next move.

It all begins with our thoughts. But what do we tend to focus on and judge harshly? Our actions—what we've done or eaten, or not done or not eaten. We focus on the behavior even though it wasn't the behavior that started the mess. Let's begin to use this formula to change things before they ever happen!

Some practical examples:

- *I can accomplish what I want to accomplish, in spite of obstacles.* This thought leads to feelings of confidence and hope. Feeling confident and hopeful leads to the courage to do things differently. Doing things differently will get you to your health goals.
- *I've already tried everything. I've tried for years. I just can't change.* Such thoughts lead to feelings of despair and discouragement. These feelings lead to the same old behaviors. There is no strength to change when these feelings are in place even though the ability to do new things is fully intact.
- *Oh no, it's Friday and I can't ever get through a weekend without gorging myself.* This thought leads to feelings of helplessness. Feeling powerless leads to the same old behavior weekend after weekend because you do not believe anything else is possible.
- *I am an active and healthy person.* This thought leads to feeling peppy and capable. Feeling this way leads to moving and enjoying life—which leads to more moving and more enjoying it—which leads to health.

This is powerful. Deciding to think and then speak to ourselves from a position of *yes* is a game-changer. Actually, it's a life-changer.

PART V

Rewriting Your Eating Scripts

Changing Mindsets and Situations That Lead Us to Mindlessly Overeat

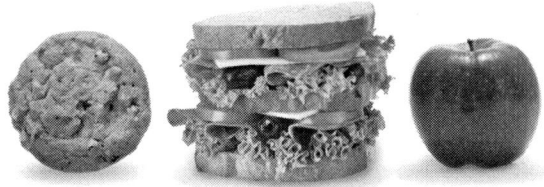

Chapter 22

MINDSETS THAT TAKE US WHERE WE DON'T WANT TO GO

Eating on the Run, Can't "Waste" Food or Money, Multitask Eating

Actors in a play follow a script—show after show—repeating the same lines in the same place to tell the same story. This works powerfully for Shakespeare or Arthur Miller because their stories are well written. But what happens when we unwittingly follow scripts that continually harm our health and sabotage our goals?

Following a script puts us on auto-pilot . . . it's been rehearsed and rehearsed until we aren't thinking anymore; we're just mindlessly eating every time we get in that situation.

The good news is that we can rewrite our scripts. Often it's just a few scripts that lead us to overeat regularly. Many people change a stubborn script or two and then begin to release the weight they have struggled with a long time.

In this chapter we will look at three of the most prevalent unquestioned mindsets and in the next chapter, situations.

Eating on the Run

One of the deadliest enemies of mindful eating is eating on the run—not just on-the-run in body, but on-the-run in your mind as well. Our full schedules can drive a frenzied rhythm of life. Relaxed time to refuel and refresh is often not even on the radar screen.

When we eat on the run we end up taking in a lot of fuel that doesn't register in the mind—but does in the body. There's never time to sit down, relax, and enjoy a meal. It's waiting until you're famished to eat, then grabbing whatever is quick and easy and eating it in the car right out of the bag while in route to the next thing.

We can get hooked on the adrenaline rush or feel that we're not accomplishing anything if we're not breathlessly busy. With eating on the run comes speed-eating, gulping down large bites, under-chewing, barely noticing you've eaten, eating it all because there's no time to recognize our "full" signal, and feeling hungry again soon because the whole eating experience is lost in the frenzy of the day.

There certainly can be something exciting about eating on the run. The problem is that there is nothing exciting about feeling heavy and slow and tired. If you struggle with eating on the run, you may find it helpful to find a quiet spot and reflect on the pace of your days. Ask yourself a few questions:

1. What is the general pace of my life right now?
2. Do I like this pace?
3. What is this busy-ness doing for me?
4. What is it taking from me?
5. What purpose is it serving?
6. How is it affecting my health?
7. How is it affecting my family and friendships?
8. Do I have a choice right now?
9. What do I want the pace of my life to look like this time next year?
10. How could I plan a little and make a big difference?

Sometimes dropping one thing from your schedule will give you the margin you need. If it's hard to tell people you're backing out of some things, you can blame it on the preservation of your health—your health requires your time and attention too.

If this chapter of life must be busy then a little preparation can go a long way in putting you back in charge of your health. Find some foods to have close by (in the car, office, purse, etc.) that will support your health and energy so you don't feel you have to run through the drive-thru often. Nuts, apples, and grainy crackers with peanut butter don't need refrigeration. Getting a small cooler for cheese, turkey, pickles, hummus, raw veggies, nut butter, fruit, etc. is no trouble. Once you get used to opening the freezer and grabbing the frozen thingy, throwing it in the little lunch box and putting some real food in it—it's really not a big deal. I was the *Drive-Thru Queen!* And I hated packing lunches for some reason. I had a mental block about it. My friend, Gwyn, made it look like a cinch, so I watched her and gave it a try. Now I know how easy it is and I actually prefer it.

One other thing we can do is decide to *slow down on the inside,* even when we can't slow down on the outside. This is reframing. Pretend there's a metronome in your core. Set it to a nice relaxing tempo. Every time it switches back to *fast,* slow it down again. Stay vigilant. Eventually your mind and body will get the message.

Be mindful of tension in your body. Is there tightness in your shoulders, your neck, your chest, your gut right now? Slow stretching and deep breathing are both very helpful for bringing peace to a frazzled mind and body. It would be best if you can find a quiet, place to do this—but take what you can get. Remember to show up and slow down at least on the inside when it's time to eat. Relaxed, mindful eating will become your new normal, even when you have a lot to do.

> We can get hooked on the adrenaline rush or feel that we're not accomplishing anything if we're not breathlessly busy.

And please, please, please realize that most of us have more control over our schedules than we admit.

How Can I Waste This Perfectly Good Food (or Money)?

We've touched on this before but it's so pervasive that it deserves another look. This mindset feels reasonable but ends in weight gain and poor health. We are often over-served, so we must learn to be at peace with leaving food behind—sometimes lots of it.

It is certainly wise to "get the most for your money," so leaving food on your plate can feel counter-intuitive, but if we stop and think it through we will realize that we're listening to old messages from the past that will not work well in the present, or we're thinking emotionally rather than rationally.

Overeating to "get your money's worth" doesn't make sense. It's like continuing to pump gas as it spills out on the pavement. You just wouldn't do that.

Think about what we're paying for when we eat out. We're paying to be nourished, for convenience, for the chance to visit around the table without preparing a meal, for food we don't normally have at home, for service, and for a certain atmosphere. Once you have those things, you've gotten your money's worth.

Eating past full—past feeling great when you leave—means the money was not as well spent as it could have been. The resulting overeating will cost a fortune in medical expenses and quality of life as the years go by.

If you're not convinced, take some time to research costs of being overweight. Look at medical costs, pharmaceutical costs, mobility issues, and quality of life issues. Getting this script rewritten will save you a lot of money . . . not waste it.

Multitask Eating

Another widespread script is multitasking—believing we can get more done if we do a lot of things at once. People eat at the desk, on the phone, in the car, in front of the computer, and while walking between tasks. They have to think hard to remember what they ate, or even *if* they ate. Sitting still and being present with their food feels foreign—maybe even irritating or undeserved or downright boring. As with eating on the run, this mindset has as an undercurrent of belief that fueling one's self and time to rejuvenate does not deserve time or effort.

Eating this way makes it almost impossible to be mindful and connected to the eating experience. When we eat like this, we often keep wanting to snack all day because even though we've eaten, we didn't *experience* the food.[14]

The ironic thing is that the person who wishes to accomplish so much will be much more productive and creative if they take a break and enjoy their meals.

Biologist John Medina, in *Brain Rules*, has this to say: "Multitasking, when it comes to paying attention, is a myth . . . research shows that *we can't multitask*. We are biologically incapable of processing attention-rich inputs simultaneously." He goes on to explain that when we do several things at once, we *feel* productive but it may take as much as 50 percent longer to accomplish tasks while making up to 50 percent more mistakes. Here's a scary example: Studies show talking on a cell phone causes drivers to be slower to brake in response to emergencies and take longer to resume normal speed afterward. More than 50 percent of the visual cues spotted by attentive drivers are missed by cell-phone talkers. And simply reaching for an object while driving increases your risk of an accident nine times.

We're discussing eating and not driving, but the same principles apply. When we eat while doing other things, we are terribly distracted and don't remember eating. And then, of course, we want to eat more.

Multitasking does not save time. Being rested and refreshed by eating a meal mindfully makes one *more* productive, not less.

If you are a multitasker, here are a few suggestions:

- Do some research yourself on multitasking. Make your own intentional decision about how you want to live.
- Consider a paradigm shift. Work when you're working. Play when you're playing. Eat when you're eating. We will enjoy (and remember) our life much more this way.
- Decide to start with mindfully enjoying one meal a day. Set your inner pace to "relaxed" and simply enjoy your food. Notice how you feel during and after the meal. Try this for a few weeks and check your productivity and satisfaction factor.

We get to choose how we want to live our lives. We can change how we have always done things. We are never stuck. When it comes to eating on the run, feeling guilty about "wasting" food or money or multitasking, each of us can evaluate and make changes that will bring more life and health into our lives.

Chapter 23

SITUATIONS THAT TAKE US WHERE WE DON'T WANT TO GO

Changing Our Automatic Overeating Scripts

S top and think a moment. Where and when do you most often over-eat repeatedly? These situations are your eating scripts. Some examples might be: grazing from ten o'clock to bed time, Tuesday night Rook club, munching in front of the TV, eating popcorn *every* time you see a movie even if you just had dinner, keeping a Coke in your hand all day, eating while cooking, always eating two plates piled high at Mama's for Sunday dinner, eating "a little something" with the kids when they get home from school, going straight to the pantry every time you walk in the door, always leaving a certain restaurant too full, automatically grabbing one of whatever is in the break room, regularly overeating on the weekends . . .

The good news is we can rewrite our scripts.

Wendy began to finally turn the corner with her weight when she changed her iced tea script. She was drinking four or five large glasses of sweetened iced tea a day. Without realizing it, she was taking in a lot of fuel. As we began to talk this through, she discovered that this was adding about four hundred extra calories to each day. Her first response was that she would just give it up cold turkey! But what's the problem with this? Our experience tells us that when we completely cut off something that we really enjoy, we can begin to feel deprived and eventually go right back to where we were—overdoing it. After looking honestly at which of the glasses of tea she most enjoyed, she decided it was the 10 a.m. glass. Kids were in school; chores were done; she had time to relax. She began to fully enjoy that glass of tea, putting her feet up and intentionally experiencing it as a gift. The others, which she drank with meals, were replaced by glasses of water. Every now and then she'll have an afternoon glass, but not regularly. This is permission at its freeing best. Wendy ended up having her tea and her health too. With our wellness vision firmly in view and a little creatively we can coach ourselves through anything!

She did have to work through some sadness at first, but it was more than worth the work when she weighed having her favorite glass of tea against reaching her health goals. And by the way, if a person takes three hundred calories out of her usual day it adds up to a release of thirty pounds in a year—without dieting.

Often just changing one or two scripts can change everything. Let's take a look at some of the most common ones and some things we can do to rewrite them.

Fun, Food, and Fellowship Scripts—Social Gatherings

Social gatherings are an overeating script for many people. And they happen often. It doesn't matter if it's friends or family, holidays or weekends, work or church, birthday parties or banquets—it's lots of food (the kind you don't have at home) and multiple distractions! In his revealing book *Mindless Eating*, Dr. Wansink and his team at Cornell found that in all the fun and excitement, it's easy to lose track of whether we've had one roll or five, four chips or forty. We just aren't paying attention. We tend to eat fast if we eat with fast eaters, slow if we eat with slow eaters, eat dessert if others do—even if we've already had it—and, in general, we eat more and longer in a crowd.

An Exception to the Rule

For those of us who struggle with food or weight, social gatherings can be exactly opposite—we may eat light in public and heavy when we're alone. This adds to our feelings of isolation, hopelessness and shame. This is part of my own story. I lived this out many times in many ways, but one moment I particularly remember happened in college. After leaving a party, where I didn't eat a bite because I felt self-conscious, I drove to Shoney's drive-in and ordered two hot fudge cakes and ate them both. Alone.

If I'd only known then what I know now. My behavior made perfect sense, but all I could assume was that I was deeply flawed and carried a terrible secret.

Please hear this. You are not flawed. If you've eaten half a red velvet cake in the grocery store parking lot, using a credit card for a utensil . . . if you've eaten an entire flat of Hershey bars and had to run back to the store for another so your kids wouldn't miss them . . . if you've gotten buy-two-get-one-free dozen donuts and eaten one dozen yourself before you got home . . . you are not alone.

Let this sink in: You are not weak or willpower-less. This behavior is shared by millions and is perfectly normal for those of us who have experienced repeated diet deprivation, thought our bodies were not acceptable, experienced a trauma that causes us to turn to food as a safe place, had a food police in our lives, used food to meet a need, lived with criticism or perfectionism or a million other isms . . . or if you just find yourself in a confusing place with food and aren't even sure why.

The truth is you can recover. You can be well. You can grow to a place where you can eat anything in front of anyone and be quite at peace. That said, the fact remains that many of us overeat in certain social settings. Let's explore how we can go to these events with tons of food, eat what we would like, and still leave feeling good. Listening to our stomach is always a good answer . . . but we will probably need other supports in place in such a distracting environment.

Here are some other ideas that will help you leave feeling good:

Concentrate on Why This Social Event Is Happening

Remind yourself what is really important to you here. Is it your neighbors, family, old friends, new ones, your nephew's tenth birthday, the bride and groom, friends from work? Go ready to savor them and the conversation even more than the food.

Try this mental experiment. Next time you're at a gathering, imagine that you are there—alone. The people have suddenly disappeared. All the food is there, the tables and chairs and decorations—everything. But not a person in sight.

I played this mental game the last time I was at our Cathcart family Christmas. We all gather in my cousin's big basement with tables and tables of great food. It's a room full of noise and energy and history and people from infancy to eighty-something. I imagined this festive occasion without my family. Just me and the decorations and all that food. To be honest, it was jarring. I felt a deep longing and earnest appreciation for these people who have known me all my life. I wanted to visit with each of them as if it were the last time I would ever see them. It really is those people that make that day what it is. The food supports and enhances, but it's not the heart of the gathering. Not even close.

Concentrating on the reason you're there, whether it's dinner with a couple of friends or a class reunion, puts the awe in its real place and food becomes a good but secondary gift to go along with it.

Talk Down Your Food Anticipation

Begin to notice your feelings of excitement or preoccupation about the food *before* the event. If you find that you're getting overly excited or anxious about it, stop and put the food in its place by speaking the truth about it. You will find what resonates with you. Here's a start.

Inner Dialogue: Talk Yourself Through

- *I am going to enjoy a relaxed and intuitive eating experience.*
- *I can have this food anytime I'm hungry. I will certainly see it again.*
- *It's just food. It's not all that.*
- *The food is not the point. I'm going to enjoy the people most of all.*
- *I can feel great when I leave this party.*

Recent research[15] can teach us a lot about our food anticipations. When people who scored high in food-addictive characteristics were told they would receive a chocolate milkshake, the pleasure centers in their brains lit up as if they had just won the lottery! When they actually drank the milkshake, the pleasure they received did not live up to the pleasure their anticipation had promised.

"It's a one-two punch," writes researcher Ashley Gearhardt. "First, you have a strong anticipation, but when you get what you are after, there's less of an oomph than you expected, so you consume more in order to reach those expectations." What can we learn from this? Remember what we know about the brain. There is the grownup and the demanding child. In the case of food anticipation, we can choose to let the grownup lead. We can decide that we are not going to let our emotions rule the day. They've ruled before, but we haven't liked the consequences.

> Food is certainly a good gift, but we cannot allow it to be our biggest thrill. Remember the level of health you desire and play your wellness vision over in your head.

We can recognize that our anticipation is out of proportion to what is reasonable and choose to change our thinking. Food is certainly a good gift, but we cannot allow it to be our biggest thrill. Remember the level of health you desire and play your wellness vision over in your head. Take a few deep breaths and repeat, "It's just food. I'm a reasonable and mindful eater. I've got this."

Use the Tools That Fit You Best

Walk in the room thinking like a discerning connoisseur, eat the very best bites first, decide before you walk in where you want to be on the Hunger/Satisfaction Scale when you leave, chew thoroughly . . . there are many effective tools (listed in Appendix C). Choose one or two and use them confidently.

 Several other helpful strategies are:
- Hang out away from the food tables.
- Don't go starving.
- Be one of the last through the food line. First ones through get seconds more often.
- Sit with the slow eaters.
- Watch "thin eaters" eat. You might be surprised by what you see. Some of them eat "thin" everywhere they go, and some eat a bit more than they usually do when they're around foods they don't normally have. There's no formula to living well with food. We will each find our own intuitive way.

Late Night Eating and TV (or Computer or . . .) Script

Recreational eating late at night is a very common script. And it makes sense doesn't it? You've pushed all day, you're worn out, work is done, things have finally gotten quiet, you're in your comfy clothes, and it's time for a mini-vacation. Time to veg out.

So, how are we going to keep our nightly relaxation routine and also reach our health goals? What can be done when the thing we enjoy so much is also the thing that is keeping us from the health and weight we will enjoy so much?

Research tell us that regardless of age, people who watch a lot of television are more likely to be overweight than people who don't. TV leads us to pay almost no attention to what we're eating, to eat automatically without asking if we're hungry, to eat too long and to sit a lot. But I think the biggest danger is that TV watching can dull our desire to do other things.

Watching TV puts the brain in a kind of mild trance. We easily forget about other great stuff we like to do, and we also don't think about tomorrow . . . as in consequences. We wake up in the morning feeling a bit hung over, try to forget the two bowls of Moose Tracks we ate last night—but our pants remind us. Ugh, not again.

Here's the deal. We all need down time. Relaxation is a legitimate need. It is also true that if we take in more fuel than we use we will gain weight, and we don't like that.

We must—and can—find a way to relax and unwind that isn't going to harm us. Let's look at some things that have helped countless people change this harmful script and turn it around.

Think Through What Will Bless You

What do you love to do besides eat? What relaxes you, entertains you, brings pleasure to you, or feels like a reward when you need one? Stop and think this through. Write down five to ten things and keep them handy. There is always a way for us to meet our true needs and have our health. Figuring this out can be *fun!*

Here are a few helpful ideas. Start a new tradition of strolling before TV time. Many people have said this really changed things for them because half the time they never make it back in for TV at all. As they walk around the block they run into neighbors, the kids start playing, it feels too good to come inside, they enjoy putzing around the yard, etc.

Keep your favorite TV nights but have three or four nights dedicated to other fun things like game night, spa night, arm wrestling night, craft night, puzzle night, art night . . . you get the idea. Start writing that book of short stories you've been thinking about. Late night gardening can be fun. An hour of night hiking is heavenly—especially in lightning bug season. Find an elderly neighbor and read to them once a week. Get books on CD and do some relaxing stretches as you listen.

The possibilities are endless! The hardest part is doing something different the first, second, and third time. After that the spell is broken and you wonder why you haven't been doing this all along. TV is so easy, so distracting, so mind numbing that it's going to take some effort to do anything else—but I will tell you that after years of coaching I have never, not once, heard anyone say that they want to go back to the nightly coma. Making these changes adds color and interest and joy to our lives and feels darn good, inside and out.

Be Intentional About What Happens Before *the Bewitching Hour*

Get your food fuel during the day when you need it. Many people don't get enough fuel during the day (the old diet mentality whispers to "eat light" or "be good") so they're too hungry by dinner time, and then dinner lasts till bed time. Eating like this can create a vicious cycle:

> . . . eat no breakfast or a snack on the run . . .
> . . . grab a light lunch . . .
> . . . feel hungry on the way home . . .
> . . . grab something quick before dinner and eat it too fast . . .
> . . . eat past full at dinner even though the snack kind of ruined it . . .
> . . . graze till bedtime . . .
> . . . go to bed feeling heavy and regretful . . .
> . . . wake up thinking you better skip breakfast since you overate
>   last night . . .
> . . . and the cycle repeats . . .

Can we just agree that this is not working?

Fuel well in the day because that is when you need fuel. Then get to dinner reasonably hungry. Choose foods that you enjoy while making sure you get enough protein and some healthy fat. Protein is the most satisfying kind of food, and fat helps slow digestion. Slow down and make dinner an enjoyable, refreshing time. Light a candle. Sit and talk for a while.

If you're eating alone, give each bite attention and enjoy a good book or magazine between bites, if you like. Make dinner an experience for yourself. When it's fully enjoyed, your tendency to prowl at night is cut way back.

Changing our late night eating script will make a huge difference in our weight struggles. Much of our overeating is done before bed. When dinner is given its due, it is very easy to be *done* and not eat again till breakfast. After dinner go brush and floss. This signals eating is done for the day.

If snacking means a lot to you, you might wish to make one or two nights a week a "yes" night and have a late-night-snack planned for. Remember, we have abandoned all-or-nothing eating. On this night, eat a light dinner and later have your favorite snack. Enjoy.

You can trust yourself with this kind of moderation once the old diet mentality is diminishing and permission doesn't push the "I blew it" button. Talk yourself through it.

Ed was really struggling with late night eating. He chose to do several small things differently and rewrote the script. He started making time for a satisfying breakfast and lunch. He had some almonds on the way home from work so he was not ravenous. He started walking the dog when he got home from work instead of immediately eating dinner. This helped him wind down and relieved the guilt he had been feeling about not walking the dog. His dog had been watching him eat dinner and the sight of his un-walked furry friend was causing him grief, which was affecting his dining experience. He determined to truly enjoy dinner and then declared "Fuel-Free After Eight." This is a guideline and not a rule, so if he does eat after eight now and then, there is no reason for guilt. This is simply a tool to remind him not to eat mindlessly and automatically. It also made him much more intentional about dinner. He also decided to go to bed a half hour earlier, which made him feel better and shortened the time he might be thinking of nibbling. The cumulative effect of these changes worked like a charm.

Here's something that helps me with grazing after dinner. If I find myself standing in the kitchen snooping around, I ask myself a question out loud. I put my fist to my stomach so I can be mindful of it and then I say *out loud,* "Am I really hungry? Do I need fuel right now?" Then I answer myself *out loud* either yes or no. I'm almost never hungry. This goofy little exercise helps me turn around and walk out of the kitchen. Getting your thoughts out of your head, into the air, and into your ears helps you hear and then think with your grownup brain. The child in my brain is the one who wants to graze most of the time.

Speaking of kitchen, I have friends who display a KITCHEN CLOSED sign on the counter in plain view after dinner is cleaned up. The sign states that the kitchen will reopen in the morning for breakfast. Clever!

If you decide you do want to enjoy something some nights, consider rethinking what you eat. Give yourself a little gift. Something interesting. Hot tea the way you like it. I'll have mine with a little sugar and whole milk, thank you. Maybe a very interesting tea cookie. Sparkling water with ¼ cup grape or cranberry juice and lime over ice is refreshing. Savor a good piece of chocolate or best fruit in season.

You May Need to Take Drastic Measures

If you find yourself still stuck in harmful patterns after trying these ideas, here are a few hard hitters. After all, drastic times call for drastic measures!

- *Change your bed time.* Stop going to bed late. This is a game changer—so simple and with so many benefits. Get in bed early enough to get eight hours of sleep consistently. This is great for your health and your food life. Fatigue is *often* misinterpreted as hunger. Sleep deprivation is clearly linked to weight gain. Go to bed.
- *Change your environment.* Rearrange your TV room. Paint it a different color. Watch from a different spot or a different room all together. Once you revamp things, declare that room a FOOD-FREE ZONE. Remember, you have a long-standing pattern to eat

in *that* room, in *that* spot, in *that* cozy chair, at *that* time of night. If we keep everything the same each night, we will probably keep getting the same results we've been getting. Changing your surroundings facilitates change.

- *Declare a TV-free month.* Give yourself room to see what you're missing. I have friends who do this several months a year and the whole family loves it (after the initial shock).
- *Kill your TV before it kills you.* If your health is in danger and change is just not happening . . . take your TV out back and leave it there for a month. It will die of exposure and you will live on in good health. Or you could donate it to a nursing home.

Take this seriously. What will happen if nothings changes about this? Play it out. One year from now, two, five, ten? This sitting and eating every night is a serious health hazard.

It May Be Time for Reflection

If you're not physically hungry but you're continuing to want to eat night after night no matter what changes you make—stop and sit with it a while. Sit quietly and see what feelings you can identify. What is behind this need to eat every night? Identify what you're hungry for: Relief? Reward? Pleasure? Safety? Entertainment because there are not enough interesting things in your life right now? Some time alone? Comfort? Distraction? Only you can know this, but you do have to take the time to think about it in order to identify it.

Please understand—these are legitimate needs. If you're a parent, caregiver, employee, business owner, volunteer, a retiree who hasn't found your next passion yet, in a difficult chapter of life, etc., you probably *do* need the things listed above. Your job now is to figure out how you can get your real needs met without losing your health.

When you just can't stop: It is possible that overeating is doing something so important for you right now that you *can't* give it up. It just keeps happening. When you have all the tools and knowledge and motivation you need and you continue to be stuck in your old eating pattern, it's time for a deeper look.

Life can bring some very heavy chapters. Food may be the equalizer for what is out of balance, medicine for a wound or a needed coping tool. If this is true—please hear me on this. You need some help. All of us need this from time to time. I certainly have. Please do not keep beating your head against the same wall. Find a trusted counselor, mentor, life coach, wise friend—get the help you need to navigate through this situation and move forward. This is a wise, necessary and courageous thing to do. I see this often on this journey. Many of us need some specific help for a time and then we can move ahead and into the freedom we were born to have.

Clean Your Plate Script

Clean. Your. Plate. Three very powerful words—words many of us heard in childhood and still influence us today. Words that override our common sense and wisdom. Words that often determine our health. These words might have made sense in The Great Depression—but in our over-served world they do not. They teach us to be mindless and work against our intuition.

"Good boys clean their plate." This was the message stuck deep within Stan's heart. He is now a grown man—successful, generous, and respected. But this statement rang loudly in his mind and greatly influenced his relationship with food, which in turn affected his health. It's a pregnant statement. His passive/aggressive mother repeated it all through his childhood and it carried heavy undertones. He got the message loud and clear. "Good boys clean their plates, and I know you want to be a good boy. If you don't then you're a bad boy. If you don't clean your plate it will disappoint your mother and we don't want that. She works so hard for you." He knew that if he ate all the food on his plate it made his mother happy which kept things more peaceful around the house. This may sound like a gross exaggeration to some, but for a child growing up with a parent who got much of their meaning from their children's lives, cleaning one's plate is serious business. Food can be a powerful tool in the hands of wounded, manipulative, or controlling people.

James tells of watching helplessly as his little sister sat at the table, unable to leave until she ate every bite—which, by the way, was put on her plate by an adult. He cringed as she repeatedly fell asleep, falling face first into her food. Still, she was not released from the table. He longed to rescue her, to eat the wretched food for her, but their angry, controlling father wouldn't hear of it.

Beth recalls the day her food-life changed course. She was about nine years old and it was the day of their big annual family reunion. A day she loved because all the cousins were in one place. At lunch time there were rows and rows of food tables piled high with everyone's favorite home-made dishes. As she went through the line, she overfilled her plate and couldn't eat all her food. She was full and ready to go play with cousins who were gathering on the lawn for games. As she was about to run to the yard, her father decided that she had to clean her plate that day. That day. Perhaps he saw disapproval in the face of an elder he admired when they saw the food still on her plate. Perhaps he felt the need to prove that he had control over his children or that he taught them the value of not being wasteful. Whatever the reason, the situation went from bad to worse as she became the center of attention—and of course could not possibly eat all that food. The cousins were shouting her name oblivious to the unfolding drama. She felt all adult eyes were on her, and her father was unyielding. The tension became increasingly thick. She felt embarrassed, ashamed, and powerless. Food became an impossible issue, a power struggle as she had to sit there until her plate was clean—while all the other cousins played. The adults watched on, probably equally uncomfortable but saying nothing. No one came to the rescue. No one changed the plan. No one brought relief or reason. I would wager that even her father wanted to call it off but felt he would lose face. This was a defining moment in Beth's life—when food went from fuel to something else, when food went from being a non-issue to an emotionally charged substance. That experience damaged her relationship with her dad, herself, and food. From that day on plate cleaning was an arrow in her heart.

These stories are heart rending and are not as rare as we would hope. They remind us to look with grace on each other. Many have come through much and could have chosen something much more harmful than food as a way of coping. When we hear these stories we can say, "Congratulations, friend. You are still standing. You have survived. And you can heal."

Healing is certainly possible! These memories and the strong feelings attached to them can lose their hold on us. We need support to do this good work—and it is so worth it. We can pull out the arrow and move forward stronger and wiser for the experience. And we can help others when we have summoned the courage to ask for help ourselves.

Hopefully the majority of us have not experienced painful stories to this degree. Many of us simply heard a steady string of well-meaning messages such as, "Eat your vegetables before you can have dessert," "Clean your plate before you can go play," "Eat five more bites and then you can leave," etc.

Most parents just want their children to get all the nutrients they can. But these kinds of statements disregard the child's inner wisdom and ability to self-regulate. These messages teach us to stop listening to our body and to eat past our natural satisfaction cue.

Not all Clean Plate scripts were formed in childhood. For some, the compulsion to eat-it-all came in adulthood as a way to "get my money's worth." Whatever the "clean your plate" statement means to you, it is time to be released from it.

Here are some helps:

- **Get excited about this!** For many of us, rewriting this script may be the only thing it takes to have the health we want. Most people begin to release weight as soon as they are free of cleaning their plate. Think how much unneeded fuel we have to store when we eat everything put before us.
- **Remember that permission works both ways.** Give yourself permission *not* to eat it all. You are free. You have permission to eat what you want and permission to leave as much as you want.
- **Open your tool box.** Use your tools over and over again until you've built a new normal: Relax, breathe, find out where you are on the Hunger Scale, become present before you take a bite. Enjoy the best bites first, pause halfway for a breather and to figure out how your stomach feels. When eating out, use the Two Plate Approach from Chapter 11. These tools work. They change things. Use them faithfully. Use them when you don't even want to and watch yourself move forward.

Eating Out

Overeating food we order is another very common script and one we must rewrite since many of us are now ordering take-out and eating in a restaurant at least five times a week. The food is tasty, it can feel "special," the first thing out is scrumptious chips or hot rolls, we're distracted by noise and commotion, and we're grossly over-served. This all adds up to a real obstacle to our health goals.

But what is the truth here? Hear ye, hear ye! The truth is we CAN leave *any* restaurant feeling great. We can accomplish what we want to accomplish in spite of chips and salsa or big, fat yeast rolls and honey butter or French bread and olive oil. Yes we can.

Let's think this through. Does overeating make it taste better? Does overeating make eating out a better experience for you? Does feeling like you need a two-wheel dolly to get back to the car make it a nice evening? No to all. We get in the car after a lovely meal and think, *What in the world! Why did I eat all that? It would have been the perfect evening if I had just stopped when I knew I was satisfied. Now I'm miserable. I told myself I was not going to do this again . . .*

When we have "done it again," we are in the perfect place to make important changes. Right then decide to be the curious observer, not the critical judge. Instead of berating yourself or just ignoring it and acting like it never happened—it's time for reflection and insight.

Sit with it a while. Relax and begin to think through the experience:

- How were you feeling before you got to the restaurant ?
- What kind of day had it been?
- Where were you on the Hunger Scale when you arrived?
- How was your anticipation factor about eating out? Were you looking forward to the evening to a reasonable degree—or too much? Had you noticed?
- At what point during the meal were you "just right" satisfied? What happened that kept you from stopping then? What if you had?
- What one or two tools might you have used that could have changed things?
- If you had intentionally relaxed and eaten at a slower pace, might you have enjoyed the very same meal without overdoing it?

Think through each step and then play through the scenario the way you wish it had happened. Acknowledge that you can make those choices next time. Remember the feeling of regret that you have right now. You may want to go back and review the two kinds of sadness in Chapter 12. You can use this unpleasant experience to bring satisfaction to your future eating-out experiences. Stumbling is a necessary part of change.

Here are some other tools and strategies for eating out and staying healthy. Pick the ones that resonate with you:

For starters, do not go starving. If you "save up your hunger," you are setting yourself up for overeating. When we are overly hungry we eat ravenously and fly right past our satisfied signal.

Plan ahead for success. Before you arrive replay your wellness vision. Remember what you *really* want. Have a conversation with yourself before you go in: *What will make for a great evening? How do I want to feel when I walk out of here? What tools will I use tonight to make this happen?*

Show up and slow down. Intentionally relax your mind and body. Walk in peacefully. Sit down with a relaxed attitude. You've got this. Enjoy each moment. When the food arrives eat in mindful mode. Being in charge of your momentum is a powerful thing. Remember your speed bumps: Drink water or put your fork down between bites to slow down the chain-chewing pace and to truly taste each individual bite.

Pay attention to bite size and chewing well. Will half that bite be just as good or maybe better? Remember that much of a large bite never hits the taste buds so a lot of good taste is wasted.

Order intuitively. What will be satisfying right now—for your health and for your taste buds? What is your body telling you? What will give you the life and energy you desire hours after the meal is finished?

Think through the bread or chips situation BEFORE you get there. What are your choices? I see at least three. I can ask them not to bring it. I can enjoy a reasonable amount while being mindful not to spoil my main meal, or if the chips are the big deal to me that day, I can make a meal of them and tip big. This is probably not a choice any of us would choose often, but it is an option and may help us get over a chip obsession.

Ask for dressings and gravies on the side. This is not because they're "illegal" but so you can be in charge of how you want to eat your salad or mashed potatoes.

Ask for a to-go box when you want one. Some people prefer to box up part of the food before they eat, some after. It's up to you. Some prefer not to use a box but to put their utensils on the plate when finished. This is a signal to yourself and your waiter that you're done. Getting the food out of sight is the goal. If it's difficult to stop eating, remind yourself that you will probably eat out again soon.

Pace yourself if you're eating several courses. Eat a few very best bites of each course. Savor lavishly. You will be so glad you did when you get to the last course.

Be reasonably informed about the amount of fuel in restaurant food. There is often a surprising difference between food we prepare at home and food served in a restaurant. Not only are the portions different but the preparation and ingredients are different as well. Sometimes the discrepancy is breath-taking. For instance, a slice of mom's homemade apple pie is around 280 calories of fuel. If I order an apple pie desert at some well-known restaurants, it can range from 590 to 960! If I have a scoop of ice cream with chocolate syrup and a homemade chocolate chip cookie at home, it might top out at about 370 calories of fuel. If I order the Chocolate Chip Cookie Sundae at Applebee's, it's around 1,600. American restaurant portions are HUGE compared to anywhere else on the globe. This is a big concern because we tend to think that what is put before us is "our portion," and unless we are mindful we will mindlessly eat our portion . . . no matter how big it is.

There are plenty of free apps available on Smartphones now that will give you this information. I use MyFitnessPal occasionally if I am eating something new to me.

Note: This is certainly not a return to the calorie counting of our diet days. This is about gathering helpful information in unfamiliar territory. This knowledge can inform and strengthen mindfulness.

Reframe your relationship with dessert. Make it about taste and not volume. You have already had a satisfying meal, so dessert is almost never about physical hunger. Consider adopting the three-to-four-best-bites dessert philosophy (notice I did not say "rule"). If, for some reason, you really want to eat more than that—order dessert for your meal. You're a grownup. You can do that.

Weekend Eating

Many dieters and ex-dieters struggle to get through the weekend without overeating, and for good reason. Because diets traditionally begin on Monday, we have an entrenched habit of overeating all weekend in preparation for the starvation to come. Certainly there are other factors as well like special weekend events and being off our workday schedule.

As I have become comfortable with the truth that I'm never going to have to diet again, and have come to trust my intuitive way of being with food, the compulsion to overeat on the weekends has disappeared. The script has been rewritten. Interestingly, though, even twelve years into recovery, every now and then I get the feeling that I need to prowl around the kitchen because it's Sunday evening. This neuropathway runs *very* deep!

If you have a diet history, pay close attention to your food thoughts starting on Friday afternoons.

Here are some helps in rewriting your weekend overeating script:

- Remind yourself that there is NO DIET coming on Monday morning—ever again. Seriously, let that sink in. It still makes me giddy!
- You can eat what you want *every* day.
- You have the same, peaceful relationship with food *every* day now. Your feelings may not know this yet, but they will as you continue to practice and talk to yourself. Mondays and Fridays are the same. Food is neutral every day.

- You are learning to be mindful every day. This will become second nature in time.
- Honor yourself, your health, and your body by respecting your satisfied signal every day. Remember that your stomach is your own personal regulator. It will go a long way in taking care of your health and weight when you listen to it consistently.

When you practice liberated eating each day of the week, your mind and body begin to relax and trust each other. Reason and moderation become the norm.

If we allow ourselves to think the "old way" about food on the weekends, it will take longer for our relationship with food to normalize. Keep your momentum up by living the same reasonable way with food every day.

A counselor will tell you that when our public selves and private selves are reasonably congruent, it is a sign of emotional health. This can apply to our relationship to food. As we are getting closer and closer to living mindfully with food every day—in front of people and by ourselves, weekdays and weekends—we can know that we are getting closer and closer to the freedom and health we long for.

PART VI

Fuel In, Fuel Out

Eating and Playing for a Vibrant Life

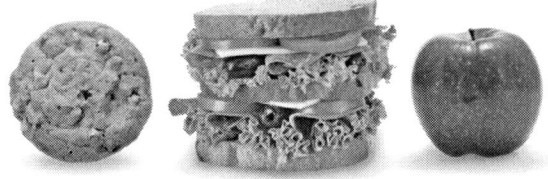

Chapter 24

THE FUEL FACTOR

The Nutrition Piece

A *note before you read this chapter: If talking about nutrition pushes your old diet-rule buttons right now, then leave it for later. It will take care of itself.*

I've put off discussing nutrition until now because dieters often see dieting and nutrition in the same light: both are about good food and bad food, foods you should eat and foods you shouldn't eat. We're now on our way to becoming liberated eaters—people for whom food is a good gift and no longer emotionally charged. This is a journey that will take some time, but perhaps we can discuss nutrition now without feeling that I'm back-peddling on permission. I assure you, that is not the case. We can eat what we want to eat. We are *not* discussing a "perfect diet," food rules, or good food/bad food lists. Period.

We also know that our highest goal is to be well. Since our fuel is a major part of this, then it makes sense to be reasonably informed. Learning how to use food to our advantage will be very satisfying.

When food is *not* emotionally charged, we can see it for what it is and make honest decisions about what we want and what will serve us well. You'll get to a place where you can choose between a juicy pear and a cupcake from a normal place of pure desire and discernment—rather than choosing the cupcake because it's calling your name or not choosing it because it is "bad."

There are countless good books and resources on nutrition. *This is not a book about nutrition*, so we are only going to hit the high spots and cover some things here that will help us reach our goal of getting well and feeling great.

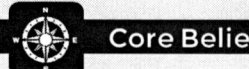

Core Belief

GOOD FUEL FOR GOOD LIFE

Since I respect my body and want to be well, I eat enough good quality fuel to thrive on.

Quick Overview of Our Fuel Needs

In order for our bodies and brains to get to do all the amazing stuff they are created to do—they need to be well-fueled. That fuel is primarily glucose. Glucose comes from the food you eat. What, when and how much you eat determines your glucose level (blood sugar level) which has a direct bearing on how you feel.

Our food consists of :

- macronutrients—fats, carbohydrates, and proteins
- micronutrients—vitamins, minerals, and phytochemicals
- water

In order to be well your body needs an adequate amount of each of these. Let's look at a quick overview:

Carbohydrates—High Energy Fuel

Carbs are quick energy fuel. They give energy fast but do not satisfy as long as protein or fat. Having an understanding of carbohydrates and your body's energy needs can make a huge difference in getting you to your health, energy and weight goals.

As dieters we have been taught to fear carbohydrates, but they are absolutely necessary for good health and are a big part of feeling energetic. There are two main kinds: simple and complex.

It helps to think of simple carbs as being fast-release and complex carbs as being slow-release.

Simple carbs are primarily fruit, honey, sugars and dairy. They are quickly digested and don't satisfy hunger for long. These carbohydrates send your blood sugar up quickly, and then down quickly as well. (Note: Dairy products contain high protein so they generally have good satiating power unlike the other simple carbs.)

Making it Work for You: Eat simple carbs with a protein rich food to give them lasting power. For example, if you eat half an apple with some nuts or nut butter or you have a pear with some cheese, you will get the quick energy you want and will be satisfied longer than if you have the fruit alone. Good to know if you need a snack to last you a few hours.

Complex carbs are primarily grains, vegetables, and beans. Complex carbs are made of starch and fiber. Starch gives you energy. Fiber makes you feel satisfied longer, helps your blood sugar rise and drop slowly so you have sustained energy, and keeps you reg'lar.

Making it Work for You: Lean toward complex carbs that are whole, that is, have not been highly processed. Processing removes much of the fiber and often nutrients too, so all you have left is starch. Without the fiber, your blood sugar will rise and fall quickly and you will soon be hungry again.

What are whole foods? Whole foods are close to their origin. They are what we've eaten for most of human history. They've not been through many refining processes. Think orange, egg, honey, fish, broccoli, grainy bread. You can picture them or their main ingredients in their natural setting and they have not changed much since then. BBQ Pringles, on the other hand, are a long way from the potato. Pringles are not a whole food.

Keep variety in mind. Eating new-to-you foods is one of the best ways to get a wider variety of nutrients and to get out of a food rut.

Whole grains, brown rice, beans, lentils, squash, peas are all great carb choices, to name a few. Try different kinds of grains for a variety of tastes and nutrients such as quinoa, barley, kasha, buck wheat, couscous, and others. I have found that they are all just as easy to prepare as the grains I grew up with and are very enjoyable.

A special note to women over forty-ish. Girls, we need less fuel as our metabolism slows down and our hormones change. This is an *Immovable*. Where we store fat can change too—often more around the middle than we are used to. Our bodies now handle some foods—especially refined carbohydrates—differently than when we were younger. Think fluffy yeast rolls, white rice, desserts, donuts and the like. I am not saying we can't eat them; I am saying we will need to adjust the quantity to fit our changing fuel needs.

> *Making it Work for You:* Many women past forty are able to reach and maintain their health and weight goals more easily if they lean toward having their high energy foods (carbs) in the high energy part of the day then enjoy proteins, healthy fats, plants and a reasonable serving of whole complex carbs for dinner. This is not hard science but I do see it work over and over again in real life.

Technically it doesn't matter when we eat our carbs as long as we're not eating more fuel than we're using, but we all know it's easy to eat past full in the evenings. We're tired. We want to chill out. There's time to relax so we tend to eat more in the evenings if we aren't mindful. Simple, refined carbs go down very easily, do not require much chewing and light up the pleasure centers in our brain like fireworks! Once we start eating them it can be hard to stop, especially at night. As always, be intuitive about this and you will find what works best for you.

This certainly doesn't mean I never have lasagna for dinner. Now in my fifties, I just adjust my portions—heavier on the salad and lighter on the lasagna than I did when I was younger. I savor the lasagna *thoroughly* and get just as much pleasure from a smaller portion as I did from a larger one. Maybe more!

> Technically it doesn't matter when we eat our carbs as long as we're not eating more fuel than we're using, but we all know it's easy to eat past full in the evenings.

Working with your body by feeding it what it needs when it needs it makes sense. We need energy during the most active part of the day. We need less energy as we gear down for sleep.

Remember, this is not a food rule. This is using what we know to our advantage. We're on a journey, and this path gets us where we want to go more easily. I have met very few women who regularly eat refined carbo-hydrates in the evenings and maintain the weight they desire—and these women are very physically active.

DIABETES HELP

If diabetes is a concern for you then it would be very helpful to do some research[16] into foods with a *Low Glycemic Index*. These are not diet foods! They are real foods that can help you normalize your blood sugar level. High Glycemic Index foods spike blood sugar rapidly, while Low Glycemic Index foods have the least effect. You don't need to eat these foods exclusively, but weeding out some of the highest and adding in more of the lowest will go a long way in helping you get well.

Protein—The Great Satisfier

Your body uses protein to build, repair, and maintain blood, muscle, and organ tissue. You also need protein to keep your immune system running well and produce hormones and enzymes. To get the amino acids your body needs, you need a variety of proteins. This is important stuff.

Protein gives the highest physical satisfaction of any food. You get protein from meats, fish, poultry, nuts, diary, soy, beans, and some grains.

Once again, *variety* is a great idea. For instance, if you enjoy peanut but-ter, try almond, cashew, and sunflower seed butter too. Rotate them for a wider variety of micronutrients.

Here are some foods with a lot of protein power: Greek yogurt, pump-kin seeds, sunflower seeds, tuna, cottage cheese, ricotta, lentils, sardines, almonds, beans, nut butters, tofu, turkey, soy beans, hummus, meats, cheeses, and eggs to name a few.

Making it Work for You: If you're physically hungry and need a snack between meals, make sure it has some protein in it so it has staying power. For example, eat a banana and walnuts, a piece of chocolate with some nuts, half an apple and some cheese or a spoon of nut butter and grainy crackers.

Starting your day with a protein-powerful breakfast keeps you well-fueled for hours: eggs, toast with turkey and melted cheese, nut butter in your oatmeal, sardines (why not?) will all keep you satisfied much longer than a Pop-Tart. If you have a serious hankerin' for a Pop-Tart, eat it with some protein.

Cereal is quick and easy but usually will not hold you for long. Less processed cereals such as Muesli will keep you going much longer than Lucky Charms. Having cereal with nuts or a spoon of nut butter for an appetizer will keep you satisfied longer than cereal alone. And remember, skim milk has no fat. If you find yourself hungry soon after a bowl of cereal you might try 2% or whole milk instead.

> *Protein is a very important part of the satisfaction-factor we're looking for from our food.*

Fats—Satisfying and Tasty

Fats keep your cell membranes healthy, manufacture steroids and hormones, regulate growth and maintenance of tissues, and keep your hair, skin, and nails from getting crinkly. Fats control appetite by regulating leptin response. Leptin tells you that you've had enough fuel for now. We want our leptin to be loud and clear!

Your body requires fats to be healthy. Without some fat we will feel hungry, deprived, and plagued by cravings. Fats make food taste good and help us feel satisfied longer by slowing down digestion. They keep foods from emptying out of your stomach too quickly.

Fat Crash Course: There are basically four kinds of fats:
1. monounsaturated fats
2. polyunsaturated fats
3. saturated fats
4. trans fats

Making it Work for You: Monounsaturated and polyunsaturated fats are known as the "good fats" because they're good for your heart, your cholesterol and your overall health.

Saturated fats need to be eaten moderately. Overeating them is linked to disease and elevated cholesterol.

Trans fats and partially hydrogenated oil are best avoided (I'm still going to have my Fig Newtons every now and then, though). Keep an eye out for products with partially hydrogenated vegetable oil listed among the first ingredients. It is primarily a preservative, not a food, and is now linked with heart disease.

Here are some ideas to help you live well with fats: Olive oil, nuts, and avocados are among the most satiating foods on the planet. Enjoy them. Wake up an avocado with lime and sea salt, salsa or balsamic vinaigrette. They are great for breakfast on toast. My friend from Brazil taught me to have them on toast with honey for breakfast.

When it comes to cooking with oil, do some research—not all oils are the same. Some oils should not be heated to a high temperature. Generally speaking, extra virgin olive oil is more for salad dressings and marinades than for cooking, at least at high temperatures.

There is a lot of conflicting info out there right now about healthy cooking oils. Just do a little research and don't get nervous about it. They'll figure it out in a few years, maybe. Meanwhile we can enjoy them using the information we have.

Micronutrients

Micro—meaning we just need a small amount

Micronutrients are small but powerful vitamins, mineral and phytochemicals.

MICRONUTRIENTS 101:

- *Vitamins (organic) and minerals (inorganic) are found in our food.* They don't supply energy like carbohydrates, fats and proteins do, but they're vital because they regulate body chemistry and body functions.

- *Vitamins and minerals, with a few exceptions, are not produced by your body.* If you don't eat 'em you don't get 'em.
- *Phytochemicals are found in plants and have important natural protective properties.*

Enjoying a *variety* of foods supports your health. Many people with food issues tend to eat a lot of the same things over and over. This decreases the likelihood of getting a wide variety of micronutrients. One of the most exciting things about our journey to becoming liberated eaters is exploring new foods.

Making it Work for You: Maximize your micronutrients by enjoying Super Foods. They are foods that pack a lot of good stuff into a small space. And they're not diet foods. They are delicious and interesting foods.

Do a little research and have fun discovering which ones you love. Consider adding one or two new ones to your menu each month.

Here is a very short list: yogurt, berries, apricots, figs, dark chocolate, eggs, nuts, kiwi, avocados, salmon, honey, green tea, oats, sweet potatoes, red beans, quinoa, spinach, olive oil, prunes, apples. Have fun researching and enjoying these power-packed foods!

TWO WORDS OF CAUTION WHEN THINKING ABOUT NUTRITION

1. **Nutritional info is constantly changing.** There is new and conflicting information coming out at a rate that will make your head spin. All we can do is stay reasonably informed, not get anxious about it, and relax and enjoy the good gift of food with our best health in mind. Getting stressed out about any of this is not good for your health.

2. **Do not trade diet rules for nutrition rules.** Both will have the same anxious, law-breaking, shame-producing effect. Remember, we are using effective tools now—not obeying suffocating rules. If you find yourself getting uptight about nutrition—leave it and go play. Please relax, trust yourself, and live!

The Western Diet

It is not my intention to tell you what to eat. This is your journey and you will find your best path. One of the many wonderful things about this liberating journey is that we are not clones of each other. My hope with this section is to give us some food for thought and the simplest of life-giving guidelines, then you decide where it all lands in your life as your journey progresses.

The Western diet is what many of us have grown up on since the 1960s and 70s. A common definition is: A diet high in saturated fats, red meats, refined carbohydrates, highly processed snack food, sweetened drinks, fast food and low in whole foods, fresh fruits, vegetables, whole grains, seafood, poultry. The Western diet has been linked to hypertension, heart disease, high cholesterol, diabetes, obesity, and colorectal cancer. Being sedentary contributes to these conditions as well.

When I think back over my childhood, there is a marked difference between food I remember as a small child and food I equate with my teenage years. I was born in 1957 and had relatives with farms and gardens. A lot of the food on the table was fresh. In the 1960's all across the country homemade food began to give way to more convenient boxed short cuts. Jell-o, Dream Whip and Kraft Macaroni and Cheese for instance. In the 70s there was an influx of prepackaged snack foods available in cellophane bags, brightly colored boxes and bottles. Chips, cookies, and candy in big bowls and abundant soft drinks appeared at every event and gathering.

Foods that had been an occasional treat became a daily occurrence.

These foods, in and of themselves, are not toxic (even though some media-hype would lead you to believe otherwise). The real problem, though, is the *amount* we eat—of anything.

Our fast and convenient foods are highly processed so much of the fiber and nutrients are gone. These foods are readily available, cheap, and designed to be irresistible.[17] It's easy to eat them to the exclusion of nutrient-rich, whole, fresh foods. We have a nutrient quota just like we have a sleep, water, activity and air quota. If we're filling up on nutrient-empty foods there just isn't room left for the foods that provide the nutrients our bodies need. If this happens then we're not going to be well—and that, after all, is what we are all about.

There are many good books, blogs and articles written on the subject of the industrialization of our food. If this interests you, Michael Pollan's book *In Defense of Food* is an interesting read. I gleaned two solid principles from this book that have stuck with me. They are simple and easy to remember—which is great in our world of information overload. Here they are, slightly adapted:

- Mostly eat food your great-grand mother would recognize as food (she would not recognize a Zinger or a Hot Pocket).
- Don't eat stuff that won't rot (very often).

Thank you, Michael. I can live with this.

So how do we make changes that stick without getting uptight or legalistic about it?

1. Don't make changes until you're ready. If you try to "eat right" before it's *your* idea, it can push the old good food/bad food button and lead to overeating in response. As the old-diet mentality dies off, the likelihood of this response will lessen.

2. When you are ready, consider making small adjustments, like adding one fresh fruit to your day. Make changes at a pace that feels comfortable to you. This process should be fun and not stressful.

3. Consider finding one "real food" alternative for one processed food in your life. You might start buying regular or steel cut oatmeal in place of instant. Keep in mind that when a food is "instant," it has been highly refined and will not have much in the way of satiating-power left. That is why you can nuke it in one minute and it's done. Other possibilities are replacing white rice with brown rice, apple sauce with apples, some snack foods with fruit and nuts. As you make small changes, other ideas will surface.

4. Keep your favorites. Decide how much of it is reasonable. Savor the smaller amount more.

5. Sometimes people are concerned about whole foods costing more. People who make this change do spend a little more on groceries but end up spending much less eating out and picking up. My workshop friends say over and over again that they're spending less and less on drive-thrus and fast food. They notice that it takes less whole food to feel more satisfied. I have never—not once—had

anyone tell me that they were unhappy with their new way of eating when they have moved in the direction of more fresh and whole food. These lifestyle changes feel good and pay off.

Here's the cool thing: as people realize they're in charge, that this is not about obeying rules, as they make room for changes in their own good time and find that they feel much more content and free—then the next natural step is to begin to trade quantity for quality, fake food for real food, fast food for slow food, scarfing for savoring, and the same old boring food for variety.

Our only question now is, "What's gonna make me feel great?" Here's Caroline's e-mail to our workshop group after a weekend of family camping:

Something crazy is happening to me and my taste buds! One afternoon I was looking around the camper for something because I was hungry. Earlier, when I wasn't hungry, I decided I wanted some of a Hershey bar left over from the s'mores the night before. I told myself the next time I was hungry that's what I will have. But when I did get hungry, that wasn't what I wanted. I wanted some protein. I didn't want to fire up the camp fire yet so I reached for the Vienna sausages, which I hadn't had in such a long time. Man, all my life I have had a thing for those slippery, delectable, bitty bites. I could slam those things down faster than I could pry them out of the tiny can. Oh, why don't I have thinner fingers? I finally wrestled that first one out, mangled, but who cares . . . first bite . . . Yuck! I better look at the expiration date. It was fine. Next bite . . . Ewwww! Did I get the wrong brand? Another label check. No, I just didn't like what I was eating! In disbelief, I had to have one more bite to be sure. No, this is junky, slimy, processed, mushy, so-called food. I wondered how it was I ever even liked those nasty little things. How did I ever eat three cans in a row once? Eating intentionally, thinking like a connoisseur, and truly being connected to my body has managed to ruin my taste buds. I think that's grounds for legal action!

Chapter 25

THE MOVE FACTOR

What About the Dreaded "E" Word? (Exercise)

hen you read that word—*exercise*—what feelings come up? If you immediately yell, "YEE HAA! Let's go!" then I'm truly happy for you. Go play and work up a sweat! If you're among those who recoil at the very idea, I understand.

David grew up in a family with athletic brothers whom his father enjoyed. He was the youngest and was kidded about being the weakling from the time he was small. He certainly was not weak, but the perception stuck and any motivation to move was smothered by ridicule and taunting. He was called lazy whenever he was caught sitting still, and he soon came to believe it was true.

Kim loved to play outside and explore. She was naturally curious, but this kind of activity wasn't acknowledged in school, so for years she just thought she was "not athletic." She was in her forties before she realized that she, indeed, does love to be active. She hikes regularly now with a cherished group of friends, and it has brought new joy, energy, and health into her life.

Katherine started dieting in the sixth grade and often went to school under-fueled. She couldn't perform well in P.E. because of this. She was naturally competitive and wanted to do well but constantly felt angry with herself for feeling weak and unable to do more. Dieting depleted her energy and over-shadowed the joy and sense of accomplishment she could have experienced.

These are just a few examples of how we can become disconnected from our natural love of play. We are all born moving and stretching and rolling around. It's intuitive. It's inborn. It's completely natural and effortless. And it's fun! If nothing had happened to convince us otherwise we would still be running, jumping, and rolling down hills and loving it.

Finding Our New Perspective

Many of us only officially exercised while we were dieting. Dieting isn't a good memory, so exercise isn't a good memory by association. Often we tried to exercise *more* while eating *less* and yet blamed ourselves for not having more stamina. Some of us burned out from *over*-exercising. Maybe exercise was your self-imposed punishment for overeating or a way to earn more food. For others it's just plain old boring. No wonder it has become drudgery for so many of us. If this is your experience, how can you feel anything other than disdain or dread?

So, how about we give ourselves a break and start afresh.

We've been reframing how we relate to food and to our body. Let's reframe how we think about exercise as well. As a matter of fact, let's just abolish it all together. If you love to go to the gym, we will cheer you on! Everyone who doesn't—you're now officially off the hook.

No more diets. No more exercise.

Separate Diet from Exercise

Diet and exercise are not like salt and pepper. They haven't always been said in the same breath. One of the biggest tragedies of the diet and fitness industries pairing diet and exercise is that too often we either do them both or we do not do either.

Because of this, through the years we've lost muscle, strength, energy, fun, therapy, stress relief, and health.

In real life *moving* is playing or working. It's natural, it feels good, and it's fun or at least accomplishes something that feels worthwhile.

You weren't born thinking moving was drudgery or that every time you ate something you should go "work it off." That's born from the old diet mentality. One doesn't earn the other. One is not punishment for the other.

Let's take back lost ground and start having fun again!

Change Your Motivation

How has exercising to lose weight worked for most of us over the long haul? About as well as dieting has worked over the long haul.

If we exercise to lose weight, we'll stop doing it as soon as we lose weight and then we'll gain it back again, or we'll get sick of doing it just like we got sick of dieting. We know this from experience.

This is an unpleasant motivation, and it won't last.

Why you want to move your body is a very important thing to figure out.

It's time to change our motivation, to focus on something else all together—on feeling great, on discovering what *you* like to do, on having some *fun* for heaven's sake, on finding something wonderful to add to your life.

> Let's reframe how we think about exercise: If you love to go to the gym, we will cheer you on! Everyone who doesn't— you're now officially off the hook.

What will happen if you begin to focus on the amazing gift of being able to move (not everyone can), on the sheer joy of stretching and bending, on the fun of playing again, on the independence your ability to move gives you, on the freedom to do what you love to do, on the power you feel, the wind on your face, the flexing of your muscles, the air in your lungs, the stress leaving your body and mind, the pleasure of breathing deeply.

Listen to these things—they are in you, they are experiential, they are about being alive, they are intuitive.

Just like *intuitive eating* is a freeing adventure, *intuitive moving* is too!

A baby is our best example of an intuitive eater; a child is the best example of being active for all the right reasons. Think of a sweaty eight-year-old boy running through the neighborhood, climbing trees, jumping in mud puddles—he's not thinking, *Man, I bet I'm building up my biceps.* A little girl jumping rope, riding bikes and playing in the tree house is not thinking, *Yea, I bet I'm really burning some calories!*

Kids move because it's fun and it just feels good—they simply can't keep from it.

Go Play Again!

Do what you love to do. If you don't know where to begin, just think back to when you were a child. Take off and find the nearest park and swing a while. It will all come back to you.

Start where you are and with what you can do right now. There is no pressure. A little leads to more. Fun leads to fun. Movement leads to movement. Energy leads to energy. Life leads to life. Just start moving . . . for the fun of it. Your activity can change anytime. You're never stuck. There are no rigid rules.

I would love to hear what you discover. My favorite play right now is hiking most days. Being outside is refreshing for my mind and my body. I also have an ancient Nordic Track and a Rebounder in the garage for bad weather days. The Rebounder, which is a baby trampoline, makes me feel like a big kid! I crank up some oldies or listen to the news and work up a sweat. For me this is play and stress relief. I recently added some small weights, push-ups (from knees) and sit-ups and am enjoying the challenge of adding more of each as I'm able.

Here's the cool thing: if it's fun to you and fits you and your life, you will keep doing it and enjoying it. Give your body a chance to enjoy being an active body and see what happens.

Paradigm Shift: If you never lose another pound, you can still be active and enjoy playing. You can enjoy being in your body *now*. And here's the irony—if you enjoy playing—you will release weight.

What if we begin to use *play* to make ourselves feel better, rather than food? Research shows it works much better!

Does the thought that you do not have to work out forty-five minutes four times a week sound too good to be true? Well, it really is true. There's plenty of research behind it. Dr. James Levine and his team at Mayo Clinic, the Centers for Disease Control, and the American College of Sports Medicine all report, after much research, that the human body can be healthy and fit without regular, rigorous workouts.

Rigid, structured exercise is not necessary for your good health. You don't have to go to the gym. You don't have to join a class. If you want to—and that's play for you—then go and love it. If not, you can stop feeling guilty.

This is *good news* for those who think they hate to exercise.

What It Takes to Be Well in These Bodies of Ours

Our intuition tells us that being sedentary is not going to cause us to feel vibrant and alive. The truth is that we are created to be active, to play and work and move. You can look at us and tell. We are primed, muscled, hinged and built for it. It's in our DNA to walk, bend, reach, push, pull, carry stuff, stretch, and go places.

Not only is being active great for the body, but it's great for the brain. John Medina writes in *Brain Rules* that after just four months of thirty minutes of aerobic activity two to three times a week, such as walking, the brain performance of former couch potatoes was greatly improved: elevated cognitive performance, memory, much less likelihood of dementia, Alzheimer's, stroke, and depression. He also says that the one factor that will determine how well we age is our level of activity. Moving and playing keeps you young in body and mind.

This Is NEAT!

In his fascinating book *Move a Little, Lose a Lot*, Dr. Levine and his team at Mayo Clinic put it this way:

> *Trying to tackle obesity through special diets and exercise . . . plainly does not work . . . Fifty years ago, there were no gyms; people rarely "exercised," and very few people struggled with their weight. We managed our weight effortlessly because we moved . . . Modern life has increasingly leeched NEAT from our existence to the tune of up to 1,500 to 2,000 calories a day. And that loss is literally sucking the life out of us. When we sit all day, our health goes into decline. Our bodies and minds desperately want to stay in motion.*

The word NEAT stands for NonExercise Activity Thermogenesis. NEAT is the calories (i.e., energy) you burn living your life. Dr. Levine defines it this way: "If you think of 'exercise' as activity for the sake of developing and maintaining physical fitness, the NEAT is everything else."

Our big problem is that there used to be a whole lot more "everything else" than there is today. Do you remember your great grandmom? I had the privilege of knowing two of mine. Monnie and Mama Norwood certainly never went to the Y or wore hot pink spandex, but both of them were lean and strong. When I think of them they are not sitting down. And they are not stressed or rushing around either. They had lives of unhurried, constant motion all day long. Standing to cook, garden, wash and hang clothes on the line. There was a gentle purposefulness about their days, and they seemed to enjoy them. There was always time to crack hickory nuts for great grandchildren or cut out paper dolls.

I do remember both of them sitting down to take a break. They would sit to enjoy some buttermilk, a glass of iced tea or a cup of coffee, but that would be about the only time they sat till after dinner. I know I look back through the eyes of a child, but I believe I am right in saying that their days were full of relaxed, directed NEAT and that they felt very well.

Our lives have changed a lot since then. Many of us sit to work and stand up to take a break. The struggle for us is that when we sit for a large part of our days, weeks, months, and years, we lose energy, vibrancy, clarity and the desire to move. Sitting begets sitting and steals the energy we were born to have. We haven't intentionally created this sit-down culture. It has evolved as our work and entertainment have gone to screens. But we can change things.

There is already a lot of discussion about change. Medical costs are forcing the conversation. As I lead workshops for corporations, I find that people are more interested and open to the idea of stand-up desks and meetings. This would have been unheard of just a few years ago.

It's easy to see that one of our biggest problems is *sitting*. The cool thing is that it's an easy fix. Much easier, I might add, than some of the crazy things we ex-dieters have done! One year I got the bright idea that I was going to get up early each morning, before the kids awoke, and roller skate around my neighborhood. This was going to be *the* answer—great exercise, something new (since I had tried everything else) and inexpensive, and I didn't even have to drive anywhere. What's not to love!

My first morning out I got around the neighborhood pretty well—even though the gravel on the side of the road almost rattled my teeth out. As I got about halfway around, I hit a section that was a *lot* more downhill than I remembered. As I began my descent I also realized that although I knew how to roller-skate, I really didn't know how to *stop* roller-skating. Meanwhile I picked up speed. The last time I had skated was the seventh grade when Dan Dejarnett and I collided in a heap, with me eventually losing a front tooth from that adventure. As this pleasant memory was going through my mind, I was still gaining speed. I'm not sure why I thought that my best option was to somehow stop mid-way down, but that was the conclusion I came to. I think I remembered that you can die on impact traveling a mere thirty miles an hour, and I was pretty sure I was past that. So I decided that sitting down was my best option. Did I mention it was summer and I had on shorts? Go ahead and clench your teeth and make that sucking sound right now. I did indeed sit down. I did indeed stop. I did indeed lose a few pounds . . . of skin off my fanny. End of story. NEAT looks very good to me.

What NEAT Looks Like

It can look different for each of us. It can fit you and your life. It does not have to be a big deal. Some of my workshop buddies have traded in their riding mower for a push mower, are now hula-hooping *with* their grandkids instead of just watching, enjoying stretching every morning and evening for ten luxurious minutes, are parking twenty minutes from work on pretty days, and swearing off elevators. I am standing up at my kitchen counter as I type this.

People have traded their desk chairs for exercise balls, talk on the phone standing up or strolling, have exercise bands and weights under the couch to use while watching TV, park *far* from the store instead of finding the closest spot, and are dancing around the kitchen while the coffee brews or the water boils.

My friends who are using stand-up desks all say they have much more energy at the end of the day now than when they sat all day. Dr. Levine's team found this to be true for them as well.

We simply are not built to sit a big part of the day. It seems that our bodies and brains are most happy when we walk about 10,000 steps a day. I bet my great grandmothers did this and never broke a sweat.

Keep in mind as you're changing your lifestyle from sedentary to active that at first it may feel like work if you've been inactive for a while. When we're used to sitting still, sitting still feels normal. But it also makes us old before our time. Sedentary people often have poor mobility as they age, feel old sooner than active people, and have a higher likelihood of memory loss—not to mention, they can't eat much without serious weight gain because they're not burning much fuel. Being sedentary is not an option for a person who wants to be well. This is an *Immovable*.

The effort it takes to change things is going to be more than worth it. Keep your health goals and dreams (wellness vision) top of mind to spur you on. Those who have adopted NEAT as a way of life say they can't imagine going back to being as sedentary as they were. They feel better and have more energy than they ever imagined and had no idea they could feel so young. No one yet has said, "Man, I wish I'd stayed sedentary . . . I miss feeling heavy, sluggish and tired."

It's important to start *thinking* of yourself as a healthy and active person. Your body will catch up with your mind. Remember, thoughts lead to feelings and feelings lead to action.

Begin looking for the most active way to do things rather than the most convenient. Make moving around a non-negotiable like brushing your teeth.

Here are just a few examples of how NEAT adjustments can make big changes in your health:

- Walking thirty minutes most days will burn an extra two hundred calories of fuel daily, which will lead to an approximate release of twenty pounds in one year. (Gender, height, and weight affect the exact amount of fuel burned.)
- Take the stairs every time you can. Six flights a day is eighteen pounds released in a year . . . and you'll have sexy legs.
- Stand to talk on the phone an hour a day and release seven to nine pounds in a year. The sixty minutes do not have to be consecutive.
- One study showed that just giving up all drive-thrus for parking and walking in for one year created an average weight release of twelve pounds. Amazing! I bet part of these results stemmed from the realization that what we think we want is not worth getting if we actually have to go in after it.

If you add several of these small things together, you'll change your lifestyle, your energy level, your pants size, and your health. Beats roller-skating downhill.

All you have to do is look at the benefits of becoming an active person and you will hop up and go play. Just take a look at all these benefits of being active:

- You get to play again
- Increases metabolic rate, which speeds up fuel burning
- Proven factor in weight release
- Better quality of life and probably a longer one
- Less hunger
- Released endorphins (natural mood lifters)
- Relieved stress
- Increased energy
- Decreased blood pressure and bad cholesterol
- Decreased insulin resistance and basal insulin levels
- Stimulated clot resorption and reduced clot formation
- Strengthened heart
- Firmer muscles
- Color in your cheeks
- Improved immune system
- Improved balance
- Improved blood lipid profile
- Reduced risk of more than a dozen kinds of cancer
- Improved brain performance in multiple ways
- Increased sense of well-being
- A natural anti-depressant
- Time alone or with others—whichever you need at the time
- A great example and benefit to your family
- An effective and natural sleep aid

Now that's some motivation and a great place to introduce another Core Belief.

Core Belief

MOVE MORE. FEEL BETTER.

My body is built to move. I play, stand, walk and move in a way that keeps me strong and makes me feel great.

For Those Who Love to Work Out

If you love to go to the gym, that's great. Go and enjoy! Remember to be intuitive about it—and don't let old diet thoughts spoil your fun. Listen well to what your body is saying so you can enjoy this for the long haul and not get burned out or injured. Dr. Levine's research makes it clear that your body is not meant to sit all day and then go crazy for one hour at the gym. Be sure to work some NEAT into your life too.

Consider Something Crazy-Fun and Way Outside Your Usual!

Fairly often I get the thrill of watching my workshop friends try something brand new and way outside their comfort zone. It opens up a whole new place in their lives. One friend bought a sailboat, the *Jessica Lee*, and has been on multiple adventures with his family. Some people have started taking dance classes who haven't danced since their high school prom in 1962. Some have bought a bike and hit the bike trails. Some people have hired a personal trainer for a period of time. Some are swimming, gardening or hiking again. Many women find that they enjoy the friendly, doable philosophy of Curves Fitness. Some have started walking clubs in their area. One friend took belly dancing lessons, for real! Let yourself go a little wild—what is it you would really love to do?

When we start this process—whatever we choose to do—a good momentum begins to build. When we move more, we feel better. When we feel better, we move more. When we move more, we want to eat less. Then we notice our clothes getting looser and our energy level increasing, and then we want to move more. This is a great cycle going in a great direction.

A Word of Encouragement for Those
with Severe Health Constraints

I have many friends on this journey who would *love* to be able to be active but have very serious health, weight, and/or pain issues. Let me encourage you. Many brave souls have made huge changes in their health and quality of life even though they started from an almost immobile place. You can improve your health and wellbeing.

Start by focusing on what you *can* do right now. Do not look at what others can do. This is about *your* health. Identify everything you can do, celebrate it and enjoy it. Tomorrow celebrate it again and do it again. Think of what is possible. One dear workshop friend couldn't walk six minutes at a time when she began moving again. She is now an avid walker.

Get some suggestions from a doctor, nurse or physical therapist. I have many friends who have found a way to join in water exercise classes several times a week because their feet, knees, and hips will not allow them to walk. Please stop thinking about how hard this might be or how much trouble. Think about the *yes*. Start thinking about where you're going to be a year from now once you start changing things.

What It Takes to Be Well

There are *so many* great books, Web sites and magazines on the subject of "exercise" so I am not going to cover that here. *Eat What You Love, Love What You Eat* by Dr. Michelle May covers the subject of physical activity thoroughly and includes an Exercise Personality Quiz to help you identify what kinds of activities you might enjoy. I hope you will enjoy doing your own research. Here we will touch on just a few things that you can implement and enjoy now.

Our great-grandparents would never have had to think about this because they were constantly chopping, hoeing, pulling, gathering, digging, thrashing, churning, etc. They also went to bed with the chickens and had no Chips Ahoy in the house, so late night eating just wasn't an issue. We live in a very different time so we do have to think about it.

Making room for these things in your life will make a huge difference.

Important Note: Make sure you check with your doctor before you start new things. It sure doesn't make sense to hurt yourself trying to get well.

Enjoy the Wonders of Walking

There's not enough room here to say it all. Getting outside and taking a walk is practically magic for your body and your mind! Fall in love with the gift of being able to walk. If you can only walk five minutes right now—do it several times a day. In a few weeks you just might feel like walking for six.

It's free. It's fun. It's simple. Walking will help get you off your meds, lessen pain, relieve stress, whittle away inches and pounds, improve balance, and reduce risk of stroke, diabetes, depression, dementia, and breast cancer. And we've just scratched the surface . . .

Get yourself one good pair of shoes and take off. Just make sure you come back.

Build Strength

As we age, we cannot have strong bones and muscles without regular weight-bearing or resistance activity. These activities build strength and keep your metabolism running efficiently.

Some ideas include: Carrying your own groceries, taking the stairs, using a push mower, splitting fire wood, using exercise bands or weights while you watch TV, hiring a fitness trainer for a season, raking, vacuuming, sweeping, walking uphill, lifting weights at home (cans of beans will do nicely), doing push-ups, digging, planting, hoeing . . .

Breathe Deeply

Breathing deeply is essential to good health. This is simple but important. Americans tend to take shallow breaths. Our sedentary lives do not require deep breathing as often as those who came before us. Watch a baby breathe next time you get a chance (remember, they're intuitive). Their little belly goes in and out, not their chest.

Here's the good news: Deep, slow breathing helps relax you, helps you deal well with stress, makes you more alert and assists in breaking down body fat.

"Five Square Breathing" is a helpful exercise I learned from Dr. David Walley. Try to find a quiet place to lie down for this. Don't worry if you don't have the luxury of lying down. I've done this while driving and still reaped benefits.

Breathe in slowly to the count of five. Hold that air in your lungs to the count of five. Release that air slowly to the count of five. Hold your lungs empty to the count of five. Repeat five to ten times.

Doing this regularly has noticeable relaxing benefits.

Flexibility Is a Big Deal

Stretching regularly relieves stress, improves balance, keeps us limber and agile, improves circulation, improves flexibility, decreases our risk of activity-based injury, and increases blood flow to muscles.

Flexibility is the one component of physical fitness that can continue to improve as we age. That makes me feel kind of stretchy and powerful.

Again, watch intuitive creatures. Babies, kittens, puppies . . . they all make a career of stretching. Try this: when you wake up, instead of flopping out of bed like a sleepy walrus and staggering to the bathroom, lay there a minute taking in the fact that you're alive. Then stretch—luxuriously, slowly, one way and then the other. Let yourself be very aware that you and your body are companions and will be all day. Become allies for an active, liberated day before you ever stand up. Stretch while the coffee brews and while you're on the phone. Stretch again before you drift off to sleep in the evening.

Swear Off Elevators for Good

Please research the amazing benefits of taking the stairs instead of the elevator. You will be shocked. It's free, and get this—it is often faster than the elevator. I have friends who have used the stairs at their home or work place to change their health one flight at a time.

Wow! There is so much more we could cover here. The main thing to know is that your body was made to move, to breathe, to be active, and to be enjoyed.

No more "should." Find the ways you like to play and go play every day!

PART VII

Balance– Gotta Have Some

Body and Soul

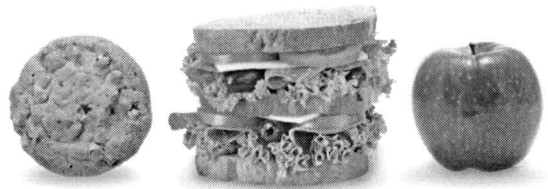

Chapter 26

FUEL BALANCE FOR THE BODY

Understanding Your Physical Fuel Needs

*W*hen it comes to food (our fuel), what does it take to get to and stay at a comfortable weight? This is a great question. We now know that it takes developing a relaxed, mindful, intuitive relationship with food—you and your body working together beautifully. This piece is a non-negotiable. After all, if our food life is causing us anxiety, we will not be at peace—even if we "get skinny" and "eat right." But what about the *physiological* fuel piece of the puzzle. Being informed about this is important, so let's unpack that a little.

Setting Yourself Up for Success

In order for us to get to and stay at a comfortable weight, here are some things to consider:

Be Reasonable

If you want to be thinner than your body wants to be, you will live in a constant battle. To maintain a comfortable and consistent weight, you and your body must agree on your "contented place." Today, with our strong media and entertainment presence, it is easy to wish to be smaller than your body and mind want to be. Please forget the "perfect" number on the scale and listen to your body. Where do you feel great? Where do you have energy and zest? You will know your happy place when you get there—if you're listening.

Wishing to be a *certain* number on the scale is dangerous. Remember Angela who released weight and went to the wedding weighing 140 pounds, feeling and looking like a million dollars? Because she hadn't reached her arbitrary goal weight of 130 pounds, however, she lost heart and gained it all back. We must be willing to be reasonable about what weight we can live with comfortably.

Be Patient

Stop thinking *fast* and start thinking *permanent*. Fast weight loss leads to fast weight regain.

This is proven experientially and scientifically. If your body releases more than about half a pound a week, it will not be "at home" in the new weight and the tendency to regain will be powerful. Many people release weight more quickly than this in the beginning, which is fine, but once the initial weight/fluid release is past and you're getting used to living with this new lifestyle, the weight release should not be fast. Please let yourself become comfortable with this. Your body and your mind must have time to get used to this new weight and fuel amount. It takes time to live and think a new way. Quick changes do not last. Period.

> Stop thinking *fast*.
> Start thinking *permanent*.

Make Both "Fuel-In" and "Fuel-Out" Lifestyle Changes

Eating and moving both matter. If we only work on eating less (fuel in) but don't learn to enjoy moving more (fuel out) it will be very hard to release weight permanently. Our metabolism slows as we age so the amount of food we need decreases with each passing year. Staying active slows down the slowing process—it keeps your metabolism young. When we're sedentary, we don't maintain muscle. Muscle tissue is a good thing to have because it burns a lot more fuel than fat tissue does.

At the same time, if you try to control your weight only by exercising but are not developing a healthy relationship with food, you are just managing your food intake by burning fuel through exercise. All it takes is one injury, illness or burnout and you're right back where you started—with a disordered relationship with food.

We don't have much choice on this one—we have to learn to eat reasonably and move reasonably. This is the way we are built.

Getting and Keeping the Weight Off—A Real Life Example

John is 5'10", 56 years old, and has weighed around 245 pounds for the last four years. Since he has a desk job and his favorite piece of exercise equipment is his TV remote control, we are going to call him sedentary at the moment. He isn't feeling great, his doctor isn't happy and John is ready to make some changes.

John's first health priority is to develop the permanent lifestyle of a liberated eater. Being the accountant type, he also wants to know about the calorie side of things. He likes doing life on a spread sheet. Here's what we figure out.

By using a Basal Metabolic Rate calculator[18] we find out that, at 245 pounds, John needs about 2,100 calories of fuel each day if he never gets out of bed. Since he does get out of bed and go to work, he needs approximately 2,500 calories a day to maintain his present weight. This is about how much fuel he's been eating each day for the past four years.

He says that he felt really good six or seven years ago when he weighed between 175 to 180 pounds. At 5'10", a 56-year-old sedentary man would need about 2,000 calories of fuel per day to maintain this weight. This is a difference of 500 calories of fuel per day. John cannot make a change like this all at once without big trouble. Here's why . . .

If you decrease your food intake by more than around 300 calories of fuel a day, your body goes into red alert. It reads this significant drop as a famine so it slows down your metabolism in order to conserve fuel. Your body and your mind feel deprived by this drastic change and you begin to crave food, especially carbohydrates since they're high-energy food. Your body will tenaciously hang onto weight in order to keep you alive and you will experience significant distress, mood changes, and anxiety. Remember the Minnesota study in chapter 2? Deprivation will lead to excess. Hyper-controlling of food will lead to obsessing over it—and here we are back to the diet roller-coaster. No thank you.

So, as you can see, just because the calculations say drop it by 500 calories of fuel—there is more to consider here than just the numbers.

As we are coaching through this process John decides that he would like to start walking. He knows he'll have more energy and it will help with his depression as well. A man his age who has some light activity three or four times a week, rather than being sedentary, will need around 2,280 calories to maintain him at around 175 pounds. This changes things significantly. Now there is only a difference of 220 calories of fuel each day. Good news.

He's very encouraged to find out that if he begins to walk three or four times a week and adds some NEAT to his day and reduces his food intake by about a tenth (eating mindfully and intuitively will make this quite doable), he is going to be able to release the weight he wants to release over the next year. No sweating it out at the Y, counting calories, or food journaling unless, of course, he wants to.

If John eats, thinks, and moves like a 175-pound person, he will eventually be a 175 person.

If he continues to eat, think, and move like a 245-pound person, he will weigh 245 pounds.

In order to maintain a certain weight a person has to find a *balance* of fuel-in and fuel-out that fits a person of that weight, height, age, gender, and activity level. This will have to become the new lifestyle, permanently, to stay at the new weight permanently.

Reality check: If we continue to eat and move like we are right now we will continue to have the weight and energy we have right now. Only permanent change brings permanent change.

It appears that the human body has to maintain a new weight consistently for three to five years before it will feel comfortably at home at this new weight. There are variables of course—like how long a person was at their heavier weight and how much and how long their weight fluctuated. It takes time to establish a new set point.

Some recent research seems to point to the body always having at least some pull back to a heavier weight. This research is still new—but it's a great reason for us to take the time to develop a way of living with and thinking about food that is sustainable, regenerative, and effective.

We must do the work of falling out of love with excess and falling in love with feeling great. Until that happens we will live in a great battle. No one, including thin people, can overeat and be well. We must grieve the loss of overeating. This is some of our most important work. And since it is painful, we will be tempted to avoid it.

For us to change, the pain of things staying the same has to be greater than the pain of changing things. Take an honest look at both pains. Only you can know which is greater for you. Don't assume you know. Stop and think it through. This is an important thing to know so you can move forward or stay put with resolve.

Possible Non-Diet Approaches for Releasing Weight or Maintaining a Comfortable Weight

This next section can be left alone or just scanned until you have walked your new eating path for quite a while. This is for consideration after the old diet mentality is mostly gone and the principles of Liberated Eating have been well practiced and are feeling quite normal.

Let's take a look at a few approaches that have worked well for some mindful eaters. As always, *these are tools* and should only be used if they interest you and work well for you. You don't have to use any of them. They are not suggestions, they are possibilities. If you try one on for size and don't like it or get tired of it, you are free to stop whenever you please. You are never trapped. If you find that you can't lay down a tool and pick up another freely then you probably have dipped back into the old diet mentality. Go back to your liberated eating basics. You are the expert on you, and only you will know what is going to be a good fit for you. I mention these approaches because I have found that over the years they have helped certain people at certain times, and it is valuable to learn from other people's stories.

> We must do the work of falling out of love with excess and falling in love with feeling great. Until that happens we will live in a great battle.

Eat to Fuel the Day, Not the Night

Maybe you've heard it said, "Eat breakfast like a king, lunch like a prince, and dinner like a pauper." In workshop we say "happy pauper." This is a philosophy I personally find satisfying. When I'm well-fueled during the day, I rarely feel like grazing after a satisfying dinner, and I'm not going to bed with a lot of food in my stomach.

Remember What Carbs Are—and Use Them to Your Advantage

We mentioned this in the section on carbohydrates, but this has worked so well for many that I think it bears repeating. Carbohydrates are high-energy fuel. Eat them during the high-energy part of the day—breakfast and lunch. Enjoy mainly protein, plants, healthy fats, and a reasonable portion of complex (slow to digest) carbohydrates for dinner.

If you're a sedentary person right now, you won't need much high-energy fuel. If this is true for you, think about keeping your simple (quick to digest) carbohydrates mainly for breakfast.

Remember, these are *not rules*. They are simply guidelines that help people keep their pants loose.

Occasionally my family likes to have popcorn for supper on Sunday night. I pop it with coconut oil. It's delicious! Popcorn is definitely a carb. On those Sunday evenings, I enjoy it fully and am grateful for it. It's just not my norm.

Become Aware of Hidden Fuel

If you don't think you're overeating but still feel stuck in the weight release department, it is helpful to figure out if you might be unknowingly consuming extra, hidden fuel. We often underestimate how much we're eating and drinking.

Take a good look at your usual food and drink. A coach, nutritionist, or dietician can help you with this if you want help. It's easy to be taking in more fuel than we think since we often don't prepare our own food. The way our food is processed has changed, ingredients have changed, and portions have changed. When I grew up, a blueberry muffin was made at home and had about 140 calories of fuel. Now most of them are bought ready-made and they have around 500. If we're not aware of this, we can easily overdo it.

Here are a few common places we can consume more fuel than we realize:

- Ordering a salad. Many fast and slow food salads contain much more fuel than one you make at home.
- Liquid coffee creamer has four times the fuel of milk. I have known people to use it like milk, not knowing that a quarter cup is like drinking a cup of milk. One workshop friend was drinking about 600 calories a day of coffee creamer and had no idea.

- A specialty cup of coffee can be around 500 to 700 calories of fuel.
- Soft drinks, power drinks, beer, or wine all have a good deal of fuel in them. Since they aren't chewed, it's easy not to think about it.
- Ordering a sandwich. Many eat-out sandwiches have much bigger bread on them than ones we make at home. I've gotten sandwiches on bread the size of a small boat. One easy fix is to make it an open-faced sandwich and eat it with a fork and knife. It's amazing how good and intentional the bites are when you eat a sandwich this way. Not near as messy either.
- Snack foods have changed a lot too. For instance, a "regular" Snickers bar is 273 calories of fuel. A King Size Snickers is 537. It's easy to think there is not that much difference—and to think you're getting more for your money if you buy the big one. Indeed, you are getting more *calories* for your money.

Looks like soon all candy bars are going to have to shrink to 250 calories or less as a regulated move toward "responsible snacking."[19]

We can be responsible right now. Stay intuitively tuned in to what works for you and what doesn't. Only you can know this for yourself.

Use Your Old Knowledge

We ought to be able to get some good out of all those years of dieting! Many of us have enough calorie knowledge to recognize what 50 to 100 calories of fuel is. We can intentionally leave about that much at some or most meals. Leaving about that much will not leave us feeling deprived, especially since we are eating satisfying foods now.

Remember that Best Bites First is a great tool for this approach because it is easy to leave the worst bites when the best ones have been thoroughly enjoyed.

Fuel Tracking (We Used to Call This Calorie Counting)

Some left-brain folks like to do the math. It fascinates them. I'm definitely not one of them, but I do have mindfully eating friends who enjoy using this tool at different times.

This approach can be especially helpful if you eat out often since there can be a disconnect to food you don't prepare yourself. This is a good way to become informed about restaurant food. Most people don't use this tool on an on-going basis. They track their fuel during a particularly distracting or busy time then leave it and come back to it as is helpful. Use it to inform and increase your intuitiveness—*not* to override it.

There are some great apps for this available now for your Smartphone. One is MyFitnessPal. I am sure there are other good ones as well.

> *Note:* Make sure this strategy stays in the position of a tool that YOU are in charge of. If it begins to feel in charge of you—drop it. An important part of this intuitive journey is being tuned to what works for you and what doesn't. Only you can know this.

> One very insightful and intuitive young woman said that every time she tries to revisit calorie counting she might as well sign a contract for a binge. This tool is not for her and she knows it.

> Another workshop friend uses the MyFitnessPal app with great success whenever she travels. She struggles to be mindful when traveling and finds that this tool keeps up with mindfulness for her. Same tool—two very different responses.

The "Yes Meal" or Treat

Some find it helpful to plan a "yes meal" to look forward to—a periodic and specific meal or snack . . . that food they've been hankerin' for.

Many intuitive eaters end up eating primarily whole food most of the time. They still enjoy a run to the ice cream parlor now and then too. I don't know about you, but this girl's gotta have her Pralines and Cream!

I have a friend who released a good deal of weight even while going with his three girls to get ice cream every Saturday. He called it Sweet Saturday. When he wanted ice cream on Wednesday, he reminded himself that he already had an ice cream date coming up.

Please understand this is not undoing permission. This is just one way that some people have enjoyed applying their permission. It's kind of the same principle as my Cookie Philosophy. I *love* cookies! Because of this I choose not to have them in my house often unless I have company to help me enjoy them—not because I "shouldn't" have them, but because I just don't want to work that hard.

Now here is the really crazy thing (and, no, I'm not just saying this): many people tell me that slowly but surely, between the freedom of permission and keen mindfulness and learning to prepare delicious foods at home, they find that their old favorites either change or just stop being favorites anymore. I have found this to be true for me as well. It's been years since I ate a slimy honey bun or those little white powdered sugar donuts or the weird ones dipped in chocolate wax—I've just lost my taste for them.

Reminder: We are far enough from the introduction to this section that I feel I need to remind you that these are merely "Possible Approaches to Releasing or Maintaining a Comfortable Weight." These are not suggestions; they are simply choices that have helped some people. Please return to the introduction if you need clarity or begin to feel pressure to try any of these methods.

Pick an Eating Style and Try It On for Size

Some liberated eaters enjoy certain eating philosophies or guidelines because it makes them feel great or works well with their particular health issues. For instance, I have mindful friends with diabetes or blood sugar issues who lean heavily toward Low Glycemic Index menus. Eating this way works best for me and my hypoglycemia. I know intuitive eaters who are primarily vegetarians or eat a Paleo menu. These people are not on diets. They are mindful eaters who have chosen a way of eating that makes them feel good—which is, after all, what we are all about. These chosen menus are tools for them, and they are free to change anytime they wish.

Some things to keep in mind if you decide to experiment with a specific menu:

- Remember that it is a tool that fits into your lifestyle of mindful and intuitive eating. Continue to be led by your inner cues—eating when hungry, savoring the food, and stopping when your body is fueled.
- Choose a menu that delights your personal pallet. Taste is part of being satisfied in mind and body.
- Choose a menu that is nutritionally balanced and provides enough fuel to keep your mind and body trusting you. Remember,

you can't take your daily fuel below 300 calories of your maintenance fuel level right now or your body and mind will feel
deprived and start the old diet roller-coaster again.

- Remember that this choice is a "want-to"—not a "should." You
  are in full control.
- Know you can stop/change at any time.
- Remember this is *not* about good food/ bad food lists, but is about
  food you have chosen because it makes you feel good and supports your wellness goals.
- Keep in mind that this changes nothing about permission. You
  have permission to eat anything. You also have permission to
  choose a certain menu if you wish to.

It is very important to understand why this is *not dieting.* The above
approaches are not about deprivation and hyper-control. You are still driven
by your body's cues of hunger and satisfaction—not rules. This will not upset
your metabolism, does not require you to weigh, does not have an "illegal"
food list—you have chosen this menu of your own free will. There are no
calories, grams, points, etc., that have to be counted, unless you enjoy that
tool. This is not an outside authority bossing you around.

These ways of finding your fuel balance are merely approaches that a
person can use to get to their best health. If at any time they begin to feel
"diety" go back and read this through and see where you might be hung up.
You are the expert on you and you are very capable of figuring out what is
best for you.

Using Your Body's Clock to Your Advantage by Getting Enough Sleep and a Twelve Hour Nightly Fast

Most of our organs have a built in clock or rhythm and the more we get in
sync with their schedule the better things work. Recent research suggests
that getting in sync with your liver by way of a nightly twelve-hour fast can
have weight release benefits.[20]

All day long your brain and body are using some of the food you're eating to power your work and play. The rest of the day's fuel is stored in your
liver as glycogen. During the night your body turns that stored glycogen into

glucose and sends it out into your blood stream to keep blood-sugar levels steady while you're snoozing. Once the glycogen is used up your liver turns to your stored fat cells and begins to burn them for energy. This is good news for those who wish to release weight!

It takes several hours to burn through the glycogen and get to the fat. Twelve hours gives your liver time to get to the fat burning stage every night. But, if we're snacking till eleven or twelve and then get up and eat breakfast around seven or eight our body doesn't have time to burn fat before we are starting the whole glycogen loading process again.

When you do happen to eat late one night it's fine to eat a late brunch the next morning so you are still leaning toward the twelve hour fast idea. Perfection is not the goal here—a good overall consistent fat-burning opportunity is.

Speaking of breakfast—it's a really good idea to eat it! To work to your best advantage, eat something with high protein and eat within about an hour of rising. The protein keeps you satisfied and energized for the morning. Eating soon after rising gives your body the signal that it's a brand new day and time to get your metabolism cranking so you burn fuel more efficiently all day. Breakfast eaters weigh less than those who skip it. Studies clearly show that people who do not eat breakfast tend to make up for it at night—night after night after night.

We know that people who stay up late eat an average of 248 calories of fuel more than those who go to bed by around 10:00. This adds up to weighing almost twenty-five pounds more than those who hit the sack earlier. Besides that, we tend to make sloppy choices at night because we're tired.

This is a good place to mention sleep. Do whatever it takes to get enough. Almost all of us need seven to eight hours each night. Sleep deprivation and weight struggles go hand in hand.

This also supports what we know about a healthy leptin response. Our leptin, the hormone that lets us know when we're full, is louder when we let our bodies refresh and repair by consistently getting enough sleep. Many people have turned their health and weight around by taking sleep seriously.

The more these reasonable practices become our norm, the easier it is to live at a comfortable weight. This is not about obeying rules. This is about understanding how your body and mind work and then using that knowledge to your best advantage.

Our bodies are unbelievably fine-tuned. As we work *with* them and not *against* them, we will come to see and feel that we are gaining strength and inner wisdom. More and more, things will begin to feel right instead of wrong.

Chapter 27

LIFE BALANCE

Understanding Your Emotional and Spiritual Needs

*W*e can't have a book about wellness without including the very important subject of life balance. After years of coaching (and living with my own imbalances), one thing stands out when it comes to lifestyle change: we can have all the knowledge, tools, and want-to—and can even make some wonderful strides—but if our lives are continually and seriously out of balance for an extended period of time, we will have an extremely hard time maintaining the relaxed relationship with food and body we desire. Food is often the equalizer, the counter-balance. It's the pressure relief valve—the way we sooth the strain of imbalance. Food is our go-to when life in the pressure cooker gets too intense.

Gaining a little more *balance* or *margin* is often the key to moving forward when we find ourselves feeling stuck. When we keep finding ourselves in the same place—returning to compulsive overeating over and over again— there's usually a very good reason. This behavior is a red flag letting us know that something is out of balance.

There may be circumstances we can't change right now, such as a care-giving situation. There may be a legitimate need that's going unmet. We all have a need for some wiggle room in our lives—for fun, relaxation, relief and down time. Sometimes it's more dramatic—like needing freedom from a toxic relationship. No one can really know this but *you*.

The problem comes when we're not finding the real answer to the real need. We often turn to counterfeits—which for us is usually food. The food can't really answer the need so we have to keep returning to it over and over again. It may numb us enough to keep us going for a while, but it doesn't solve anything.

We can even be so busy or disconnected from our true needs that we don't acknowledge that we have any. But if they're there, we cannot eat them away.

You can grit your teeth, stiffen your upper lip, put Post-it notes everywhere to remind yourself what you are about, swear you'll never eat another bag of chocolate chips before bed again . . . but . . . if there's not a reasonable amount of margin in your life, food will continue to be your counterbalance.

And you'll continue to be frustrated with yourself and your health goals.

Bottom line, you can check with any therapist worth their salt and they will tell you that every person has some unavoidable needs. If they go unmet, you will find a way to meet them or you will temporarily find a counterfeit to relieve the stress of not having them met.

These needs fall into several categories. In a nut shell, you need:

1. to know that you are safe;
2. to feel loved, to belong;
3. personal power to create, participate, and have your own opinions;
4. some plain old fun—some R & R; and
5. the freedom to be yourself—to make your own choices, take your own risks, and to be fully engaged in life.

A counselor would call the last one self-actualization. By the way, an important part of freedom is being reasonably comfortable in your body.

People who study us say that one or more of these five needs going unmet is why many of us are struggling with food or some other habit, issue or substance.

We cannot kid ourselves. If we have chronic stress or chaos, releasing weight and keeping it off will not be easy, for many reasons. One big reason is that food is quick relief—and you really do need relief, as surely as you need air.

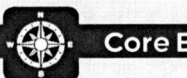 **Core Belief**

BALANCE—GOTTA HAVE SOME

I am a whole person (not just a body), therefore I nourish, exercise and rest my mind, soul, and body in a way that brings balance and health to my entire being.

All Three Parts Need the Same Three Things

If this subject resonates with you, then let's take a closer look at what we can know about building more balance. There are a few things we can examine that will help us identify where the leak might be.

It is commonly accepted that we are mind, body, and soul (spirit). All three of these aspects of ourselves need the same three basic things in order to thrive. Nourishment, stimulating activity, and rest. As we're looking for the most stable, balanced position from which to live we can use the simple triangle to help us get a good look at ourselves and our needs. The triangle is the most stable of all shapes, by the way.

Food, Nourishment

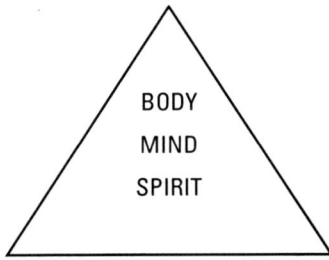

BODY
MIND
SPIRIT

Rest, Sleep, Quiet   *Activity, Work, Play*

All of us would agree that the human body needs fuel, physical activity, and sleep to be high functioning or balanced. But it's easy to overlook the equally important needs of our mind and spirit. They don't often collapse as visibly as our bodies do.

It is just as true, though, that the mind needs food for thought—or, rather, thought for food—stimulating activity, and to have some quiet time to reflect. And every soul needs to be nourished by what is transcendent, to be actively challenged to grow and stretch, and to have some peace.

Our body, mind, and soul each hunger to be fed well, to play and work, and to get some rest. Any of these longings can be mistaken for food hunger (or trigger a craving) if we are too busy or distracted to discern what the real need is. Certainly *perfect* balance is not possible or necessary—but we cannot expect to live sanely with food if some major areas of our lives are significantly out of balance continually.

> When our legitimate needs are reasonably and genuinely met, many of our cravings will stop screaming to be fed.

When our legitimate needs are reasonably and genuinely met, many of our cravings will stop screaming to be fed.

If this has struck a chord with you, consider finding a quiet spot for reflection and asking yourself some questions. Good questions can open up space in our lives for helpful ideas to be revealed. Here are a few for starters (you will think of others):

- What do you do for play? How often?
- What part of your day is quiet (no radio, phone, etc., in sight)?
- What is the first hour of your day like? And the last?
- What part of the week is your Sabbath? (This may not be a religious Sabbath for you, but when do you get to be "off"?)
- What is the most interesting thing in your life right now?
- What is a great joy for you right now?
- How often do you get to enjoy truly stimulating and challenging conversation?
- How much TV do you watch? What percentage of your down time is this?
- When is the last time you took a stroll in the moonlight?
- How often do you enjoy music?
- How much sleep do you get each night?
- When is the last time you read an enjoyable book (not a self-help book or some other required reading)?

- If you are a person of faith, how do you express it?
- When was the last time you belly laughed?
- What inspires you?
- What are your hobbies, interests, missions or passions?
- When is the last time you tickled someone?

Hopefully these questions can get the ball rolling. You are perfectly capable of figuring out what you're hungry for besides good food.

Balance is a big subject, but we are brave enough to tackle it.

I have the privilege of belonging to a book club of stellar women who love and challenge me. One evening Barbi White, a seasoned and respected therapist, made this statement:

> *Our bodies are always trying to heal,*
> *Our minds are always trying to balance,*
> *Our spirits are always trying to lead.*

This is profoundly encouraging. Just look at what is always trying to happen for us . . . healing, balance, and good guidance. These thoughts are extremely hopeful and remind us that we can trust the way we are made. Good momentum is waiting to happen as we begin to work *with* our body, mind, and spirit and not against them.

This approach to life and health is intuitive, mindful, regenerative, and life-giving—and absolutely possible for each of us.

Indeed, dear fellow sojourner, you really can accomplish what you want to accomplish in spite of your obstacles. And please know that you are not alone in this worthy quest.

Your liberation awaits!

Next Steps

Thank you for spending so much time with me in these pages. I know what you've read is a lot to think about, but let me encourage you to:

- Take a deep breath and relax. You can do this.
- Remember this is a process. It doesn't have to happen all at once. Take one good step at a time.

- Trust yourself.
- Find the support you need for the journey. This may be a trusted friend, life or wellness coach, walking partner, support group, counselor, audio workshop (available early 2013) and support messages on The Liberated Eater Web site, health professional, etc. You may want a combination of these on your team.
- Look over the table of contents and find the parts you want to revisit—you do not have to deal with this all at once.
- There are handy references at the back of this book.
- Begin to build your own Wellness Library if you haven't already. This book might be your first entry! You will find a list of good books in the back and at www.theliberatedeater.com.
- Take a walk and have fun developing your wellness vision as you go.

Thank you for the high privilege of sharing this conversation with you. Fare forward, voyager! I am praying for courage and freedom as you go.

ACKNOWLEDGMENTS

My gratitude overflows!

This book bears the mark of many people. I am profoundly grateful for each one.

To my publisher, Dan Wright; and my editor, Kyle Olund. You guys are amazing. Thank you for the comfort level you've afforded me to write this book and for your expertise in crafting a book that is far above anything I envisioned. Thank you!

Much of this book was formed in the safe womb of workshop which would not have been possible without that first brave pilot group. Thank you dear Kay, Kate, Janice, Charlotte and Mary Martin.

Deep thanks to each one who has journeyed through workshop. What an honor to have shared that sacred space and time with you. I am ever yours.

Thanks to Ray Hill—original creator of our first name, WhyWeight (and hot dog soup).

Big thank you to all who volunteered time and talent in the earlier years to give (then) WhyWeight its face: Shayne Schroader, David Hobbs, Chris Forte and David Neal.

Many more recent thanks to Lauren Murrell at Volacious Creative Media, Rob Blackford at Design 615, Melissa Thompson at MWT Media and Bill Seaver of MicroExplosion Media. And of course, to my patient computer doctor—Rick Milewski.

Big thanks to Jason Elkins and his amazing team at Transparent—for your patience, creativity and innovation. Jason, Mailynne, Ricky and Cody—you rock!

Thank you Cali and Nyk of Cali Ashton Photography, for making me laugh.

Many thanks to Ray Cleek, Jason Gibson and the friendly staff at the Babb Center and warm thanks to the FMC team: David Meyer, Jeff Lake and the happy staff and volunteers. You all provide the perfect climate and spaces for change to take place.

Deep gratitude to David Ask—you picked me up when I was down for the last count one fateful day. I will never forget the return of hope He brought through you.

Gratitude and admiration to Kay Arnold, Melanie Lowe, Barbi White, Ted Klontz, David Walley, Deb Poland, Bob Norwood and Tony Dallas for sharing your expert knowledge and wisdom.

Joyful gratitude to my soul-encouragers. You know who you are. Your dear friendships breathe strength into me over and over.

To Kay, Christi, Sharon, Kate and Em for constant feedback through this process. You are patient women.

My hat's off to you Kay Arnold. It is off and in my hands.

Thank you, dearest Immortals. Thank you.

Many thanks to Lora O'Steen and our brainstorming crew: Carol, Beth, Angie, Sherry, Laura, Chad and Christi.

Thank you to Joanne Jackson, Stacy Gammons and the good folks at Pinnacle Financial Group—for believing that this organic message could be effective in the corporate environment.

Admiration and gratitude to WellCoaches Corporation and their stellar instructors.

To all who spend their lives sharing this good message of Intuitive, Mindful, Intentional, Liberated Eating through books, blogs, research, etc. Blessings on you and your noble work. As we continue the mission may the collaborative effort cast the message far and serve to change and free many. My ultimate goal is to see the eradication of overeating so the money now spent on weight loss can go to the enslaved and underfed. May it be so.

To the amazing students, parents and tutors of The Academy for bringing it home to me over and over again that learning together is a sacred experience.

To Daddy, Mom, Stacy, Jess and the gang. You sustain and refresh me.

To Monner, who taught me that a slice of cake could be small and very enjoyable.

To my ever encouraging children, Kate, Em and J. Your deep love of Life and Truth keep me honest and eager. Gosh, I love you!

To Bob, my good man, fine husband and best friend. You are my stability, my safe place, my partner in adventure, my love. Thank you for never getting weary of this—even when I did.

And above all, to my Father—for the unfathomable way You put us together. You are Life and Light to me.

Apart from the names mentioned here there are many who mark me and this work. I can't name them all for want of space. Many have contributed to my understanding and longing to share this message. Thank you for your inspiration.

CORE BELIEFS AND BEHAVIORS OF LIBERATED EATERS

These Core Beliefs are a concentrated guide for the principles that lead to a life-giving food/body "world view." The order and the wording are not magic; feel free to rewrite them in your own words and add your own thoughts.

The deeper we get these health-giving core values into our lives the freer we become to put our food anxieties behind us and walk on in health and freedom.

Find your way of adopting these beliefs. Put them on note cards, your phone or desktop, post-it notes on the mirror . . . whatever it takes.

1. ***Being well is the goal.*** I eat, drink, play, work, move and rest in a way that causes me to be well. My goal is to thrive, rather than weight loss alone. (Chapter 6)

2. ***Ditch the diets.*** I want a healthy relationship with food, not a restrictive one. I do not diet because diets are unnatural, unnecessary and ineffective. Dieting upsets the peaceful balance that is meant to be between my mind and my body. (Chapter 2)

3. ***Listen to your body. You can trust it.*** I can trust my body. It is built for high performance. It knows what it needs, when it needs it and

how much. I pay close attention to my body's signals, such as hunger, fullness, thirst and fatigue and I honor them. (Chapter 2)

4. **Wait for true hunger.** I listen for hunger and answer it because that is when my body needs fuel. If I eat when I do not need fuel my body has to store that food as fat. (Chapter 8)

5. **Eat what you (and your body) want.** I give myself permission to eat what I want. There are no illegal foods. Since I want to feel revitalized after I eat, I choose a variety of foods that will satisfy my taste buds and energize my whole body. (Chapter 13)

6. **Listen for "satisfied" and honor it.** My body knows how much food it needs. The just-right amount of food is very satisfying. I often pause half way through my meal to "listen" for satisfaction and I stop eating when my body tells me I am no longer hungry. (Chapter 11)

7. **Enjoy each bite.** I enjoy my food. I sit down to eat it, making sure I am fully present. I have a relaxed posture, take reasonably sized bites and chew slowly—savoring the good gift of food. (Chapter 14)

8. **Handle emotions without using food.** I can deal with my emotions without using food. Food is the best solution for hunger. It is not an effective solution for stress, boredom, happiness, anger, etc. I am very capable of finding appropriate solutions. (Chapter 17)

9. **Fire the critical judge.** I am a curious observer, not a critical judge, of my eating behavior. I do not allow negative, self-condemning thoughts which keep me from moving forward. I have learned to be merciful with myself, even when I do not make the best choices. I learn from these missteps. (Chapter 20)

10. **Good fuel for good life.** Since I respect my body and want to be well I eat enough good quality fuel to thrive on. (Chapter 24)

11. **Move more. Feel better.** My body is built to move. I play, stand, walk and move in a way that keeps me strong and makes me feel great. (Chapter 25)

12. **Respect your body.** I respect my body and am very grateful for it. It is my constant companion. I have stopped wanting it to be perfect and I now value my body as it is. (Chapter 21)

13. **Balance. Gotta have some.** I am a whole person, not just a body; therefore I nourish, exercise and rest my mind, soul and body in a way that brings balance and health to my entire being. (Chapter 27)

CORE BEHAVIORS OF LIBERATED EATERS
(Chapter 7)

This is it, clean and simple. Nothing more.

1. They eat when they're physically hungry (not emotionally hungry).

2. They choose what they would like to eat with both pleasure and health in mind.

3. They eat mindfully, enjoying the eating experience.

4. They stop eating when their need for fuel is satisfied.

HELPFUL RESOURCES FOR YOUR WELLNESS LIBRARY

This is the tip of a very liberating iceberg. This short list will get you started on your own journey of finding what resources resonate with you.

Liberated Eating

- *Intuitive Eating*, 3rd Edition, Elyse Resch and Evelyn Tribole
- *Eat What You Love, Love What You Eat: How to Break the Eat-Repent-Repeat Cycle*, Michelle May
- *Eat What You Love, Love What You Eat with Diabetes*, Michelle May and Megrette Fletcher
- *The Fat Fallacy*, William Clower
- *French Women Don't Get Fat*, Mireille Guiliano
- *When Food is Love*, Geneen Roth
- *Eat, Drink and Be Mindful*, Susan Albers

Play, Activity, Fitness

- *Move a Little, Lose a Lot*, James Levine

Effects of the Food Industry

- *Mindless Eating*, Brian Wansink
- *In Defense of Food*, Michael Pollan
- *The End of Overeating*, David Kessler

Change

- *Brain Rule*, John Medina
- *Change or Die*, Alan Deutschman
- *Changing for Good*, James O. Prochaska, John Norcross, and Carlo DiClemente

Healthy Relationships

- *Boundaries*, Henry Cloud and John Townsend
- *The Assertiveness Workbook: How to Express Your Ideas and Stand Up for Yourself at Work and in Relationships*, Randy J. Paterson
- *Mind Over Money*, Ted Klontz and Brad Klontz
- *Daring Greatly, The Gifts of Imperfection, I Thought It Was Just Me*, Brené Brown

Help for Eating Disorders

This book is primarily for those who struggle with disordered eating. The list below is for those struggling with a possible eating disorder. The difference between the two can sometimes be a fine line. Thankfully there is effective help for both.

- *Bulimia: A Guide to Recovery*, Lindsey Hall and Leigh Cohn
- *Body Wars*, Margo Maine
- *The Golden Cage*, Hilde Bruch and Catherine Steiner-Adair
- *Life Without ED*, Jenni Schaefer and Thom Rutledge
- *The Secret Language of Eating Disorders*, Peggy Claude-Pierre
- *Surviving an Eating Disorder*, Michele Siegel, Judith Brisman, and Margot Weinshel

Web Sites, Paper, and Blogs:

- "Sexual Abuse, Shame and the Unintended Consequences of Obesity" by Gwen Moore (Unpublished paper, 2012, permission by the author.) To request this paper contact Gwen Moore at gwen.moore@Vanderbilt.Edu
- The Center for Mindful Eating Library: www.tcme.org/library.htm
- Wellcoaches Corporation, www.wellcoaches.com (if you're interested in finding or becoming a wellness coach)

There are many good blogs out there. If you're interested you can putz around a find some that speak your language. Here's The Liberated Eater blog and another that I've enjoyed:

- www.theliberatedeater.com
- www.canyoustayfordinner.com

Appendix C

TOOL BOX FOR BUILDING A LIFE-LONG LIBERATED FOOD-LIFE

These strategies and behavioral tools are powerful change agents. Many of the behavior changing tools are marked in the book with a tool icon: 🛠. Some strategies and "thought resources" are not specifically marked.

Coaching Note: As a coach I sometimes hear people express concern over not moving forward as quickly as they wish. After some discussion it becomes apparent that they know about the tools but are not actually using them. **To be effective these tools must be used put into practice, not just studied as theory.**

When you look into a master's tool box you see tools of all kinds. Some are well worn from frequent use. Some are used less but are valuable in certain situations. And a few are unused. So it will be with this list. Use the ones that benefit you, and create your own.

Check In Before You Dig In—figuring out if you're hungry or not, and how much (Chapter 8)

Hunger/Satisfaction Scale (Chapter 8)

Best Bites First (Chapter 11)

Two-Minute Mid-Meal Pause (Chapter 11)

Two Plate Approach when eating out (Chapter 11)

Showing Up—Setting the Stage for Mindfulness (Chapter 14)

Showing Up—Arrive Before the First Bite (Chapter 14)

Slow Down & Savor—Relaxing Your Eating Pace (Chapter 14)

Thinking Like a Connoisseur (Chapter14)

Take a Picture of Your Plate Before & After—(Chapter 11)

Relaxing Your Eating Pace Tools (Chapter 14)

Standing Firm Against External Cues to Eat (Chapter 15)

Fork in the Road (Chapter 16) for Emotional Eating

Importance Scale from 1 to 10 (Chapter 4 & 15)

Fuel Free After Eight (Chapter 23)

Kitchen's Closed Sign (Chapter 23)

Social Gathering Strategies (Chapter 23)

Late Night Eating Strategies (Chapter 23)

Eating While Watching TV Strategies (Chapter 23)

Cleaning Plate Strategies (Chapter 14 and 23)

Weekend Eating Strategies (Chapter 23)

Eating Out Strategies (Chapter 23)

A List of Possible Non-Diet Approaches for Releasing Weight or
    Maintaining a Comfortable Weight (Chapter 26)

NOTES

1. The term *intuitive eating* was coined by Elyse Resch and Evelyn Tribole when they wrote their groundbreaking book, Intuitive Eating, in 1995. It is now in its third printing.
2. *Switch: How to Change Things When Change Is Hard* by Chip Heath and Dan Heath, 144.
3. Noll, S.M. and B.L. Frederickson. "A Mediational Model Linking Self-Objectification, Body Shame, and Disordered Eating." *Psychology of Women Quarterly* 22 (1998): page 625.
4. You will find a list of tools and strategies in Appendix C.
5. If you're a research junkie you will enjoy the newly revised third edition, *Intuitive Eating* by Evelyn Tribole and Elyse Resch. Their Summary of Intuitive Eating, page 292, will give you plenty to chew on. Research abounds which points to mindful, intuitive eating being highly effective for weight release, better health and higher life satisfaction.
6. Dr. Brian Wansink, *Mindless Eating*, page 46.
7. Adapted from *Discover Mindful Eating* by Megrette Fletcher.
8. I normally would not use the word "fattening" since the real issue is wellness, but here it fits since many of us have spent much of our lives thinking food is fattening.
9. Federal Trade Commission. "Marketing Food to Children and Adolescents: A Review of Industry Expenditures, Activities and Self-Regulation." A Report to Congress July 2008. Kaiser Family Foundation. "Television Food Advertising to Children in the United States." 2007.
10. *Interesting side note:* After using this tool for a while a few people I know have come to the conclusion that they are actually satisfied with their present reasonable weight and good health. They are well (verifying this with a physician is wise) and upon honest reflection realize that it is more important to them to be able to live with their present fuel intake than it is to release more weight. They begin to be happy where they are, caring for and enjoying their body as it is. Be willing to take the time to reflect and to be honest about what is truly most important to you so you can reach your goals *or* stop struggling with this food/weight thing and enjoy this life you have.
11. See Helpful Resources for Your Wellness Library (Appendix B).
12. For much more in-depth brain info read Drs. Ted Klontz and Brad Klontz's book *Mind Over Money*. Sometimes we respond to money the way we respond to food. If that resonates with you, this would be a great book to have in your library.
13. Stanford University. Technical University of Lisbon and Bangor University and published in the *International Journal of Behavioral Nutrition and Physical Activity*. Augustus-Horvath and Tracy Tylka, 2011 Ohio State University, *Journal of Counseling Psychology*.
14. "Once eating is under way, the brain has a key role to send out a signal when fullness is approaching. If the mind is "multitasking" during eating, critical signals that regulate

food intake may not be received by the brain. If the brain does not receive certain messages that occur during eating, such as sensation of taste and satisfaction, it may fail to register the event as "eating." This scenario can lead to the brain's continuing to send out additional signals of hunger, increasing the risk of overeating." Stephanie Vangsness, R.D., L.D.N., C.N.S.D., Brigham and Women's Hospital, affiliate of Harvard.

15. Study appears in the Archives of General Psychiatry, lead author is Ashley Gearhardt, a Ph.D. candidate in psychology at Yale University.

16. The American Diabetes Association is a good place to start your research.

17. *The End of Overeating* by Dr. Kessler is an interesting book on the food industry and hyper-palatable foods created to be irresistible.

18. A dietician, nutritionist, nurse or wellness coach can help you with this. You can also find calculators online and figure it out for yourself. They all give slightly different answers so remember to relax and be happy with a ballpark figure. We are NOT going back to calorie counting. We are merely wanting to understand our own fuel needs like we understand other numbers such as blood pressure or cholesterol.

19. Companies such as Mars have signed on with Partnership for a Healthier America to shrink the size of snack foods.

20. This section is based on recent research by Dr. Satchin Panda and colleagues of Regulatory Laboratory, Salk Institute, published in the journal, *Cell Metabolism*; by Kelly Baron and Kathryn Reid at Northwestern University's Feinberg School of Medicine and by Phyllis Zee, MD, medical director of the Sleep Disorder Center.

Come Visit Us @

www.TheLiberatedEater.com

WHERE YOU'LL FIND HELPFUL FREE STUFF SUCH AS:

- *Weekly e-mail encouragements on Mondays and Fridays:* Just let me know and I will add you to our long list of folks who receive short encouraging e-mails twice a week to keep them on their intentional journey.

- *Blog posts:* Join in our blog conversation. Visit every Wednesday to read a new blog post, or sign up to receive it in your in-box each week.

- *Quarterly newsletter:* The Liberated Eater Newsletter comes out every three months or so with helps, recipes, testimonies, etc. E-mail Cindy@TheLiberatedEater.com to sign up.

- *Shared stories:* Knowledge is important, but real-life stories are inspiring! You can read stories of others on this journey and share your own if you like.

THE LIBERATED EATER
WORKSHOPS AND SUPPORT

WORKSHOP FACE-TO-FACE: Join a workshop in the Jacksonville, Florida, area. Cindy leads workshops in person—small groups, large groups, and corporate workshops.

AUDIO WORKSHOP: The 12-week workshop will be offered in an audio format for the first time in Spring 2013. You can experience the workshop in your own space and on your own schedule accompanied by *The Liberated Eater Workbook* and weekly personal work.

AUDIO SUPPORT LIBRARY: You will find a growing audio support library for those who have completed the workshop. Each week a few messages are added. You can listen as you get ready for your day, drive, prepare meals, etc. Each message is designed to support your journey, answer your questions, and provide new information and research.

And you'll find other things as well! Please share your ideas with us. We are always changing, trying out new things, and open to ideas that will help each of us on this journey toward a balanced and healthy food-life.

For more information, contact Cindy at:

Cindy@TheLiberatedEater.com

or

(615) 330-8884

CPSIA information can be obtained at www.ICGtesting.com
Printed in the USA
BVOW022126180613

323652BV00012B/345/P